"Rainbeau Mars is a health astronaut who will help you chart a course into the universe of optimal wellness."
—Robert Krochmal, M.D.

"Rainbeau Mars looks great and if you're like me, you'll try anything to look great. So why not give this program a shot."
—Joan Rivers, comedienne, author, TV host

"There is a solution to covering our mirrors and letting out our pants, a centimeter at a time. The antidote lies within Rainbeau Mars's brilliant book, an illumination of her life and commitment to personal and global health. To follow this star-lit path is to learn how to cook and eat deliciously; to flex your body-temple in breathtakingly loving ways; to cleanse the toxic and inhale the beautiful. Just think. In twenty-one days, after following this 'rainbow path,' your inner and outer self will be aligned with the 'true self' that you are. This isn't only a journey of a lifetime: it is the journey to life."
—Cyndi Dale, author of *The Subtle Body: An Encyclopedia of Your Energetic Anatomy*; *The Intuition Guidebook*; *Kundalini: Divine Energy, Divine Life*, and fourteen other bestselling books on energy medicine

"Rainbeau inspired me to have a natural childbirth (now twice) and to appreciate the power of natural health, beauty, and fitness through healing, delicious foods. I am grateful to call Rainbeau one of my best friends and teachers and excited that now, you will also."
—Josie Maran, supermodel and CEO, Josie Maran Cosmetics

"Rainbeau is very knowledgeable when it comes to healing your body through whole foods and yoga. I highly recommend anyone embark on the journey of cleansing with her program."
—Leonor Varela, actress

"In Sanskrit, yum is the mantra that opens the heart. Rainbeau Mars reaffirms that with her unique approach to peace, love, and healthiness: just some of the ingredients that make up the yumminess that is Rainbeau Mars."
—Jason Mraz, singer, healer, hallelujah

"Rainbeau is her own billboard. She truly walks her talk. This program's results are almost overnight and at times overwhelming. I encourage changing your life and giving this cleanse a try."
—Esai Morales, actor

"Rainbeau's three-week cleanse program is truly a fresh start, and I'd recommend it to anyone. She cares for her students and wants to see all of us be our very best; for that, I am so grateful."
—Blythe Metz, actress, writer, producer, ecoentrepreneur

"Rainbeau is medicine for the soul."
—David DeLuise, actor, filmmaker, father

"The 21-Day SuperStar Cleanse is a great book, and the recipes are great. A gift, really. I love how Rainbeau presents her subject matter in a positive, easy light so that everyone can embrace the ideas and start to move the needle to a healthier lifestyle."
—Ashley Koff, R.D.

"Rainbeau Mars offers a sparkly, radiant, colorful path for illuminating one's inner and outer self through nourishment in all its forms—food, yoga, self-care, and wholesome living. Light up your life with the dazzle of the superstar cleanse!"
—Dr. Deanna Minich, health expert and author of Chakra Foods for Optimum Health and The Complete Handbook of Quantum Healing

"Rainbeau Mars is the rare gift in a teacher: able to lead by instruction, example, and inspiration. I love everything Rainbeau does ... why don't we all give this program a try as well?"
—David Duchovny, actor, filmmaker

"In a world of people who don't walk their talk, Rainbeau Mars is a refreshing soul who emanates her life's purpose by simply being herself. With The 21-Day SuperStar Cleanse, she brings together a full program for body, mind, and spirit that is easy to follow and addresses the real needs of people and makes it possible to do! A beautiful book from a truly beautiful person."
—Madisyn Taylor, founder DailyOM

"Rainbeau Mars is an extraordinary yogi, actress, nutrition expert, and model, a real-life superhero."
—David Wolfe, author, health, eco, nutrition, and natural beauty expert

"Rainbeau is a teacher's teacher, brilliant, beautiful, and divinely inspired."
—Dr. Light Miller, N.D., author, doctor of Ayurveda

"She comes in colors, and she is everywhere. Rainbeau Mars is not only a yoga master of masters; she is a superstar goddess healer. She has greatly made my experience on earth more blissful. You can get it if you really want it."
—Gregory Cipes, actor, musician

"The new you is waiting. Put aside the foods that pollute, destroy, and harm, and eat what the mother has provided us—food that's healthy for your body and the planet. Rainbeau will show you how."
—James Cameron, filmmaker, environmentalist, deep-sea diver, director of *Avatar*, *Titanic*, *Aliens*

"Rainbeau has greatly inspired our family to better health at the deepest level—health and sustenance that connects the dinner table to Mother Earth and a kind of bounty nearly lost in our society. Her message is inspired, relevant to all and comes with love and wisdom. We are so thankful for the contribution she has made to our lives."
—Heather Rae, academy award nominated film producer, and daughter Johnny Sequoyah, star of NBC's *Believe*

"I've had the pleasure of working with Rainbeau and the honor of calling her my friend. Her cleanse is a wonderful way to start a happy, prosperous road to health."
—Alison Eastwood, actor, director, animal advocate

"Rainbeau is a tireless champion of spirit and all of the things that help us live more fuller, balanced and powerful lives."
—Jason Olive, actor

"With the same passion and talent Rainbeau has for acting, she has created a program to discover your potential and live a better life. This is a no-brainer—must try."
—Lewis Smith, actor, acting coach, founder of Actors Academy

"In an over-medicated society, we too often forget the ancient dictum, you are what you eat. Rainbeau Mars has offered an invaluable service in reminding us to be conscious of what we consume on a daily basis, and thus determine who we choose to be. Part cookbook, part yoga-guide, The 21-Day SuperStar Cleanse offers holistic healing that will keep the doctor away."
—Sean Stone, director, producer, cinematographer, screenwriter, actor

"Rainbeau reminds us that our bodies are sacred, and we thank her for generously offering her knowledge on the art of nourishment."
—Avasa & Matty Love, devotional singer-songwriters

"Rainbeau brings forth a new consciousness about healthy food and nourishment with this cleanse. In contrast to all the transgenic and toxic food in the world, she honors the philosophy of Hippocrates that food is thy medicine."
—Juan Ruiz Naupar, creator of Pneuma system and Inkarr, and Ciela Wynter Ruiz, U.S. Inkarri coordinator and co-creator of Pneuma Yoga

"To transform the health of the body is only meaningful if its true goal is to transform the mind and spirit of the being it houses. It is this pure intention that sets Rainbeau's technique apart from so many other healing programs."
—Ben Lee, singer, songwriter

"As the healthcare debate rages on and the costs of institutional medicine skyrocket to unsustainable heights, Self-Care is our way through the madness. Rainbeau Mars presents a transpersonal practice in luminous health and well being. The best insurance you can buy."
—Mathew Engleheart, co-founder of Cafe Gratitude and Gracias Madre restaurants

"Wherever you are in your life, taking twenty-one days to invest in YOU and your health is an extraordinary step to take, and Rainbeau makes it easy every step of the way with The 21-day SuperStar Cleanse. What an awesome way to jumpstart your journey to a healthier life!"
—Robin Berzin, M.D.

"Rainbeau's twenty-one-day cleanse is a generous way to nourish and uplift yourself and those around you. It is about abundance. It isn't about starving yourself. Her easy instinctive energetic personality takes you through the twenty-one days without a struggle."
—Ione Skye, actress, director

"Rainbeau Mars has spent her entire life dedicated to health and wellness. Her sincerity provides a shining example of how to live a superstar life with radiance that is accessible to all. Her programs allows us all to share in her secrets."
—Felicia Tomasko, Editor in Chief, Bliss Network, LA Yoga Magazine

"Rainbeau embodies health and vitality. Her guidance is practical, inspiring, and full of heart. She is a cheerleader for all people to live happy and healthy lives. And she derives great joy from the wellbeing of others. Rainbeau's ability to be both a master and a student is reflected in her practice and philosophy. We love Rainbeau!"
—Sarah and Ryland Engelhart, artists, owners, and co-founders of Cafe Gratitude

"Rainbeau Mars is a great example of natural beauty inside and out. She has inspired me to practice more yoga and lead a cleaner, nourishing life filled with joy and deep gratitude."
—Donna De Lory, singer, songwriter

THE 21-DAY SUPERSTAR CLEANSE

The 21 DAY SUPERSTAR CLEANSE

*a rejuvenating lifestyle program
to help you feel younger, healthier,
and ready to rock the world!*

RAINBEAU MARS

Creative Director: Anthony J.W. Benson, injoicreative.com
Cover Design: Anthony J.W. Benson, Lindsay Sánchez, and Anthony Scalvi
Book Design: Anthony J.W. Benson and Lindsay Sánchez

Covers and interior photos by Jeff Skerik, rawtographer.com, except as noted below.

Additional photos: Candy Hom (85); Marcomayer (105); Juan Moyano (152); Viktorfischer (175); Gary Arbach (199); Ingrid Balabanova (219); Nilsz (223); Joao Virissimo (253); Sean Macdiarmid (276); Torsten Schon (297); Antonio Mirabile (320); Rmarmion (321); Bert Folsom (325-top); Marek Uliasz (325-bottom); Irochka (331); Marilyn Barbone (334); Arrow (344); Marius Jasaitis (358 to 359); Krzysztof Slusarczyk (365)

Independent photographers: James Wvinner (21, 239); Jolie Kinga (22, 29, 71, 196); Eliza Balis (51, 151); Mikki Willis (61); Richard Salazar (89); Jessica Unamuno (117, 163, 309, 314, 318, 324, 329); Leelu Morris (129, 259, 267, 305, 330-top, 333, 335); David Paul (140); BLive (157); Rainbeau Mars (169); Alexandra Westmore (206); Kameko Kali (217); Amir Magal (292); Craig Cameron Olsen (341)

Edited by: Debra Evans and Sheridan McCarthy
Printed in the United States of America
ISBN-10: 0-9857152-1-9
ISBN-13: 978-0-9857152-1-2
Library of Congress Control Number: 2013955182
Published by: Deeper Well Publishing and Rainbeau Mars Omni Media

This book is dedicated to Mother Earth and the greatest

embodiments of Her that I have known …

my earth mother, Brigitte Mars,

my godmother, Light Miller,

the Incan priestess Dona Maria, my grandmother Rita Smookler,

and my beloved daughter, Jade Mars.

We are meant to glow and shine
It's not about ego, but what is divine
The addictions and distractions are not who we really are
I believe that *you* are meant to shine like a star
It's not about what, but how we can obtain such a goal
It's about us returning home so that we can be whole

To create peace between body and mind
Let go of what's old
Consume beauty and life
Rather than fear and mold

I see you
I support you
I celebrate you

I love the way we are, when we are being authentic
Strong, practicing boundaries without the need to protect,
The times when we reflect what is perfect
In compassion, health, and beauty, may we all connect

It is time—right now
That we exist in the possibility of the Tao
What are we waiting for anyhow?

We can illuminate on the inside
Let ourselves be virtuous and enjoy the ride
There is nowhere to run and there is no place to hide
Within our own beings, a universe resides

Come on, superstar
We know who you are
You're here, you've opened this book,
So let's take a look
The secrets you are looking for
Are within every cranny and nook

It's not the distance or how far
It's bringing light to the dark that lets us *be* who we are
We are perfect beings of light; this is our birth-right

We know the difference if it's serving us or not
Is it making us blocked, afraid, or hot?
Are we aligning with our goals or just living like sloths?
We can have everything we ever wanted
Positivity can reclaim the addiction that's taunted

We have everything we need to be healed
To let who we really are be revealed
A better fate sealed

I am you
You are me
We are worth it

The key is to focus on the heart
If it is coming from the head, it acts out of habit and forces us apart
The time is now
Everything we ever really needed to be the stars
It's time for us to raise the bar

Sit back and enjoy the ride
Allow me to humbly be your guide
With my heart on my sleeve
Your health the intention
This is nothing new, but there will be rejuvenation, ascension

Together we can be the most glowing
Examples of our brightest selves
With our past on the shelves
Walk with our heads high
And let love attract to us
Be patient and self-realized in faith and in trust
Change is constant, but come it must

If not us, then who?
We already know what to do
If not now, then when?
Let's visualize love, beauty, abundance, and Zen
Think of this as an inner galactic tour
So that we become "the ones we've been waiting for."

CONTENTS

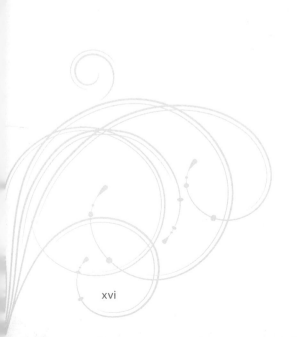

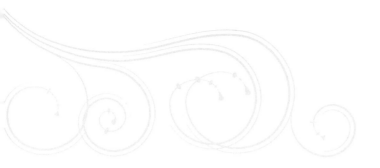

FOREWORD

I met Rainbeau Mars when she had just come of age; I believe it was the ripe old age of eighteen. I was playing Larry Flynt in Milos Forman's movie and eating live foods to operate in peak form. It was on the set of that movie that I got to know and truly appreciate Rainbeau's being. She was surprisingly comfortable on a three-day shoot for a scene that turned out to be her first in a feature film, and one that ended up in the trailer, no less. Milos and my brother and I all had an instant connection with the young beauty.

Rainbeau brought a refreshing glow to the set down in Memphis, the kind of iridescence that her name implies. I believe that her clear and abundant energy helped her stay centered in herself and confident in her ability to handle all the new people and experiences. For example, I was struck by how comfortable she was in her birthday suit, which is not so easy for the majority of actors. Now I understand how that was an early indicator of the way Rainbeau would choose to live and work in the future—willing to bare heart and soul for the sake of what she is passionate about. And I can tell you, Rainbeau is passionate about off-the-charts health.

On the set, I remember her sipping fresh raw juices and knocking on my trailer for sprouted bread. We shared an appreciation for superfoods before the name even existed. I was moved when Rainbeau told me she wanted to contribute to the world in the ways that I did—spreading the word about health, the environment, family, freedom, and love—because I knew that she meant it and would do just that.

I adhere to the information in this

book and wholeheartedly support Rainbeau in

sharing her wisdom with the world.

It has always been a pleasure to cross paths with Rainbeau in the years since that first meeting, whether at a rainforest fundraiser, rollerblading at the beach, or sharing spontaneous moments of dancing, fun, and song under a canopy of stars with friends in Hawaii. Wherever she goes, she brings an aliveness and an openness to life that I admire. I have watched Rainbeau do the opposite of what many young people do when they come to Hollywood: instead of losing herself in the matrix of games, she actually found herself—a testament to her character.

She now has a yoga and live foods center and is doing exactly what she intended—making detoxification, healing, and health a rich and meaningful adventure. I was surprised when she told me that I had inspired her immersion in yoga, but if I had any part in it, I am proud of that. She is a naturally inspiring teacher, and her yoga style is fresh, intuitive, and evolving.

I adhere to the information in this book and wholeheartedly support Rainbeau in sharing her wisdom with the world—a knowledge of health that has turned into wisdom by *living* it every day. This twenty-one-day program she has developed as a day-by-day guide for achieving greater health and happiness is the real deal. If you let Rainbeau take you by the hand, you will feel better in one month than you can imagine right now.

Beyond the personal benefits to be found here, I think it's valuable to see this program in its larger context. Rainbeau's work is also a response to the global emergency that is taking place right now, from eighteen billion animals being eaten for our consumption to global warming and oil spills. As the saying goes, if we are not part of the solution, we are part of the problem. We are each being asked to awaken and take responsibility for our health and the health of our planet. Like my wife and me, Rainbeau is raising her child in harmony with nature and humbly doing her part to serve the healing of our global family.

I believe that Rainbeau Harmony Mars is part of the solution. She treats the body like a temple to be honored and the earth like a garden to be loved. And her approach to inspiring others to do the same is offered in the pages of this book with clarity and care.

In Green Health,
WOODY HARRELSON

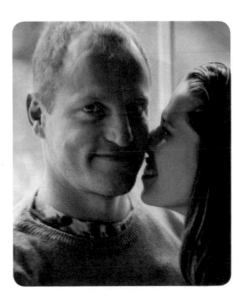

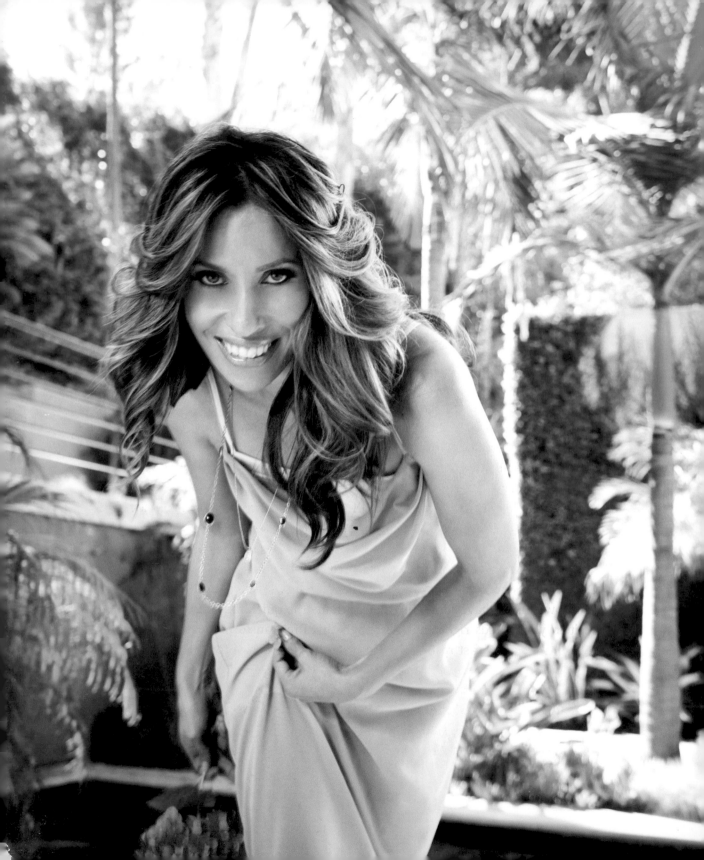

INTRODUCTION

When you open your eyes in the morning, do you feel a surge of excitement or a quiet sense of optimism about what the day may hold for you? Are you propelled forward by a certainty that you're either living your dream or you're moving toward it? A wise mentor of mine says, "Your future should be more exciting than your memories." But I know that for far too many of us, that is simply a nice sentiment. It takes *energy* to get excited, or at least to sustain that excitement. Sometimes we're hit with bouts of fatigue just when we need to be at the top of our game. Or we're plagued with health challenges that prevent us from even being in the game at all. I have had so many friends and clients plead with me, in so many words saying, "Rainbeau, just give me the quick fix. Show me how to feel good again—no, to feel *great* again!" And you know what? I have something better than "the quick fix," and you're holding it in your hands right now. Although this life-transforming three-week process does offer fast results, it also provides a blueprint for a lifetime of radiance. For years I myself have been doing this program before I step on set in front of the camera or embark on a teaching tour. It's the Fountain of Youth that my friends and clients have claimed for themselves so they can look like, feel like, and *be* superstars in whatever they do. But it's an inside job; the magic and charisma are to be found within oneself.

I remember a first intention-filled meeting with a dear friend who became a client, a wonderful woman who was completely exhausted by her efforts to feel better and "fix" things from the outside. She had changed her hairstyle, makeup, clothes, accessories, and car. She regularly got facials, body wraps, hot stone massages, and other spa treatments. And yet as delicious as each of those things is, none of them gave her what she was really seeking. The sparkle had gone out of her life, and she was slowly giving up. As she talked about the private suffering that she'd been enduring, we cried together … but not for long, because she committed herself to *The 21-Day SuperStar Cleanse* process and reclaimed her vibrancy and passion—one day, one healthy bite, one deep breath at a time. She became completely luminous, with greater ease and pleasure than she had ever imagined.

AND NOW IT'S YOUR TURN. IT'S YOUR TIME TO SHINE.

To start with, you could think of this program as a kind of time-release supplement that does its magic over the course of twenty-one days. In the space of three short weeks, you will be resetting your system and discovering how quickly your body responds when you nourish it with whole, living foods. As you support your body at a whole new level, you will also be amazed by how quickly it responds to your attention and kindness.

Throughout the pages of this book, I will be at your side as you discover how rapidly the inner transformation can take place. And beginning right now, you can let any ideas of restriction or limitation just melt away, because what I have in store for you is a bounty of delicious, rejuvenating foods and new activities that will prove to you that radiant beauty, health, and indulgence can and do coexist. Over the years, I have become what I call a passionate "flexitarian"—someone who is more interested in enjoying a wide array of abundant, delicious, and enlivening foods than advocating a dogmatic set of rules to follow. Although the specifics of the program are laid out for you step-by-step in the chapters ahead, at the heart of the matter, *The 21-Day SuperStar Cleanse* offers foods that regenerate and ideas to re-create; it's about giving your body and mind a refreshing time to reset and restore, offering clarity and balance. And it's about making choices that will help you to feel totally alive and beautiful for the rest of your life.

This program provides a fresh start for your body, mind, and soul, and I am excited to support you in discovering how easy it can be to feel radiantly alive and fully aligned with your ultimate potential. I am devoted not only to supporting you to reach your health and beauty goals, but also to discovering—or remembering—the things that make your heart beat faster, the quickening that comes from putting your attention on whatever it is that calls you to your greatness. And if you commit yourself to the process, you are about to have more energy than ever before to actually heed that call!

My passion for this program of renewal comes from a place of empathy, of understanding the pain of feeling separated from myself, rejecting my life purpose, and getting caught in cycles of food addiction and sometimes abusing substances like cigarettes and drugs, as I did during periods of my younger days. And like many people, for a long time I didn't realize that the solutions were right in front of me (or if I did, I definitely did not apply them until it became necessary). This has surprised some of the people around me, given the type of upbringing I had. I was raised along the foothills of Boulder, Colorado, by an extraordinary woman, Brigitte Mars, a master herbalist, respected holistic health educator, author, and now a raw food chef as well. My mom instilled in me a deep sense of connection to the planet and a knowledge and respect for the medicinal power of herbs and whole foods. Little did I know then that my childhood would provide the solid foundation in natural health that I would come back to as an adult and continue to build upon. Like many young people, I had to seek and find my own way, which included a fair amount of rebellion against my earthy roots. My stepdad was an interesting fellow, and when he kicked me out of the house (starting at fourteen) I would go live with other people and find ways avoid the pain I pretended not to be in. Thank goodness one of those moves sent me to Hawaii, where I lived with Ayurvedic/chiropractic doctors Light and Brian Miller, and an island yoga and healing education went into full bloom.

After high school (I graduated at seventeen) I spent time living in Europe and Miami and explored modeling, which was not my passion. I received my first movie role around that time in Memphis, called *The People vs. Larry Flynt,* starring Courtney Love and Woody and Brett Harrelson. I moved to Los Angeles to pursue my career and turned nineteen shortly afterward with my new Hollywood buddies. The LA casting experiences were many and difficult, sending me into self-judgment and self-sabotage and a need to make peace. I remember eating pancakes, pizza, cookie dough, Doritos, cookies, and muffins, drinking lots of milky, sweet chai, smoking cigarettes, and then starving myself (even working out at midnight) before jobs or auditions. It was a yo-yo I could not sustain forever; something would eventually need to give. Woody and his brother Brett sort of took me under their wing and brought me to a Power Yoga class. The first time I experienced the sweaty, kick-my-booty, crowded-room-with-the-sweet-calm-feeling-afterward type of yoga, I became hooked. They also had me read a wonderful book called *Fit for Life.* Later Woody and Dr. DeAndrea would open a live food and herbal tonic restaurant on Sunset called Oxygen that was my hangout. These were the grounding things that kept me connected in between my studies and grand pursuits in the oh-so-chaotic city. And although it didn't happen overnight, yoga and healing foods gradually became an unexpected refuge, teaching me a sense of balance, presence, and happiness in the midst of the wild temptations and self-doubt that Hollywood can lend.

When I began practicing yoga on a regular basis, I realized that I was undernourished, physically and emotionally. As I gradually started paying attention to the neglected parts of my body and inner being, there was no avoiding the depletion I felt. I quit my regular modeling job at Sebastian and began to place my attention on what was inside me rather than outside. But there were some trials and errors. For one, in an attempt to feel more grounded, I got into macrobiotics—and gained twenty pounds, not being used to so many grains and yogurts and eating regular meals. I ended up feeling too grounded … literally weighed down. But perhaps that's what I needed at that time to get myself onto the mat and delve into deeper dimensions of myself. As I breathed, stretched, and felt my way through my yoga practice, sadness and tears came to the surface. Years of abandoning myself could no longer be suppressed, and I began to realize the immense pressure I had put myself under in the pursuit of my young dreams. For an entire year, I cried at least twice a day. As the tears flowed, I felt the stirrings of inner guidance letting me know how much was as stake and what I stood to lose if I didn't learn to love myself.

To stay internally focused, between auditions I took on the job of folding blankets and cleaning up the yoga studio where I practiced, which was owned at that time by two of my beloved teachers, Maty Ezraty and Chuck Miller. I will never forget the day that permanently altered the course I was on. Chuck walked over to me as I stood in the middle of the studio with a broom in my hands. In the way a wise teacher can pose a question as though opening a combination lock to your inner self, he simply said, "What is Rainbeau here to do?" The response that came from somewhere deep inside my being was:

I think I'm here to love myself enough to inspire others to do the same.

And that was it. I chose to take teacher training to deepen my understanding of what there was to unravel, get more than an hour-and-a-half workout, and in turn, I suppose, heal my soul (although I would not have used these words at that time). That was the demarcation point when I began sharing yoga on the side with those who asked me to and found that another world of education had opened up to me, even as I continued my pursuit of work as an actor. Although the parts I was up for felt shallow and at times difficult, there was a breath of fresh air in my life from serving up health, connection, and yoga. I will always be grateful for the doors that opened to a path that I would not have predicted.

It was at Woody's daughter's birthday party on Maui that I discovered the true meaning of "having my cake and eating it too"—and found it such a delight! The gorgeous Renée Loux made a raw birthday cake, and it was like a light switch got turned on. I finally took up the famed (and in my eyes wild) Juliano Brotman, author of *Raw: The Uncook Book*, on one of his many offers to teach me how to stay beautiful and healthy. I was planning a birthday party, and I wanted to "have my cake and eat it too." The pioneering raw food chef wasn't subtle in his insistence that I try out the raw vegan diet. He eventually moved into my home (the balcony really, as he slept only outside) and immediately poured out my boxed almond milk to make sure I only ate raw. He shared incredible food from his—at the time—underground restaurant and taught me how to prepare live, enzyme-rich meals. As I ate this way, my body felt more alive than I could remember since childhood. Old knots of tension simply unraveled. I soon met Jules's friends like David Wolfe (the live food superhero and author of *Eating for Beauty* and the life-changing *Sunfood Diet Success System*), author and teacher David Jubb, and Juliano's then apprentice Matt Amsden (owner of RAWvolution). There was never a dull moment.

Living on a high-raw food diet, I noticed an astounding difference in my yoga practice and overall health. Synchronicities increased and I continued to manifest people who steered me on this path, including Jeremy Safron, author of *The Raw Truth*, and my beloved Schatz brothers on Maui, Ethan and Eli, who climb coconut trees, and like their buddy Woody, only run their vehicles on recycled cooking oil. As I continued to have my eyes opened with live foods, I noticed that other aspects of my life seemed to come together magically, even effortlessly at times. Something inside was different, and rather than the all too familiar low-grade fog I felt from unhealthy foods, I experienced a continuous stream of creative ideas, inspiration, and love, all leading to an abundance of new opportunities.

My success rate on booking the jobs I was going out for became ridiculously high, and I also received multiple requests to do yoga DVDs, although I kept acting and turned down the first nine requests. I didn't realize I was meant to teach yoga, since that was never my intention. Finally I accepted my first job to film four videos on Maui (the Hawaiian vacation was the hook for me), and seeing Molokai in the distance was especially confirming. How I had gone from being a confused student (hiding under a hooded sweatshirt) in the back of class to creating my own yoga DVDs was a little strange—but something I breathed into and accepted, learning what I could from it all. Acting parts started to pour in at an uncanny pace, but I found myself pregnant and another story was about to unfold: giving birth to my greatest teacher, my daughter, Jade.

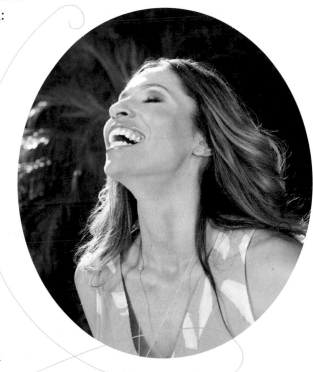

As I think many of us discover, the different paths of our lives often converge at some point. For me, my acting career and my journey of self-discovery with yoga and living foods began to merge with my study of meditation, martial arts, and authentic seeking for connection to the unseen. I am more grateful now than ever for the countless gifts I learned from my mother and other blessed teachers, each of whom have inspired the work I do today with

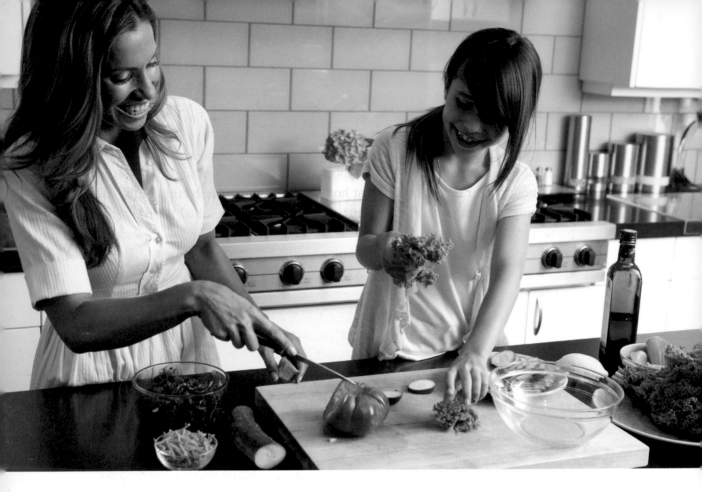

people around the world. It seems funny and wild to me that I have now created countless DVDs to help support people's health, beauty, and fitness. But it's true what John Lennon said: "Life is what happens to you while you're busy making other plans" … and I love being of service. *The 21-Day SuperStar Cleanse* program evolved naturally as I was sought out by people who were looking for a way to transform their health and appearance that was manageable and effective. Living in Los Angeles, I have worked with many actors, models, musicians, and others in the entertainment industry who often need fast, noticeable results—often to lose weight and amp up their charisma for movies, photo shoots, and concert tours. As fun as it is to support creative people in preparing for their projects, some of the most rewarding consulting has been with people working to release an addiction, heal from an illness, or assist with prenatal and post-pregnancy nutritional support.

Becoming a mother myself is another influence on this program, as having my daughter and watching her grow have truly brought my purpose into focus. Although a California girl at heart, I moved to the Caribbean islands where Jade's dad had grown up for what I thought would be an ocean birth. Instead, Jade's underwater birth happened at home in an Aqua Doula birthing tub. The experience was amazing. Despite thirty hours of back pain, I had the energy to persevere, and birthing itself was painless and drug-free—which I attribute in large part to eating a mostly live food diet. As I see Jade flourish with health, confidence, and happiness, my dedication to helping others discover boundless health simply increases. She's a child whose favorite foods are kale salad, seaweed, and gluten-free pasta. Her teachers say that she is unusually compassionate and the strongest girl in her class, and I know that this is everyone's birthright. The light that emanates from my daughter is something I also see returning to so many of the people I have the privilege of witnessing on this journey of health and virtuous living, whether individually or in groups.

Boundless health is not meant for children only; nor is undimmed light. They are meant for you too, whether you are thirty years old or ninety-five. You can reclaim them by wholeheartedly taking this three-week journey with me. In essence, this program offers tools for discovering and aligning with your ultimate potential: for embodying your destiny rather than escaping it. Integrating the best of what I have learned and shared for more than a decade, I will walk alongside you through these steps of clarifying what you want and discovering that having it begins on the inside. In other words, what you want is right at your fingertips. *The only work to do is internal.* Deeply nourish your body with foods, thoughts, and feelings that wake you up and everything else will follow. The job, the adventure, the experience, the lover, the opportunity—it will come. In fact, you can use this cleanse process periodically to keep strengthening different aspects of yourself. I do it myself seasonally (and sometimes more often), and I will tell you, if there is something you want, this program is the hookup! I've seen this time after time with my friends and clients. As you come together on the inside, the outer world will reflect that back to you in ways you will love. This, I promise.

ONE OF MY PASSIONS IS TO HELP YOU
GET YOUR HEALTH IN LINE SO YOU CAN
DO WHATEVER YOU LOVE ... AND WITH A
LITTLE MORE FAITH AND EASE.

This program has been my saving grace and always gives me back even more than I put into it. One distinct example is the three years I spent as the global yoga ambassador and consultant for adidas. Each month I traveled to a different country and needed to arrive ready for photo, video, and TV shoots, meetings and media interviews, and to teach large classes where my handstands needed to be solid and my backbends deep. With the toll of traveling and the time it took to create content and work, I actually had less time to practice, and this program saved me every time. Without fail, it always got me exactly where I needed to be, energetically, mentally, and physically.

Whether I'm preparing for a role, a shoot, or a wedding, this program works every time, and I am grateful that all I need is twenty-one days! I assure you that I love to relax, eat, and chill like the best of them, but my passion for being my best for what I love always keeps me coming back, and it's so much easier than living a life of restriction or lack.

I INVITE YOU TO COMMIT TO AND ENGAGE
IN THIS TWENTY-ONE-DAY PROCESS
WITH AN OPEN MIND AND HEART.

Page by page, you will be given the structure, guidance, and support to make your journey through the three weeks fun, revelatory, and ultimately successful. I've designed it to be manageable for everyone—moms, husbands, executives, students, and jetsetters alike. With daily menu plans, affirmations, virtues, environmental ideas, and recipes to focus on, you will have exciting choices to undertake. A daily dose of yoga—focusing on both classical yoga postures and samples from my integrative fitness system known as *ra'yoKa*—will help you ease into motion.

There are many ways to grow and transform, but I can say without hesitation that the simplest way to go about it is this program. Consuming amazing food while practicing positive affirmations and virtuous living will roll away any inner cloudiness that may have gathered, allowing your inner light to shine. We must let go of who we've become so we can be who we are.

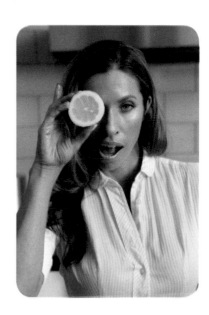

RAINBEAU MARS

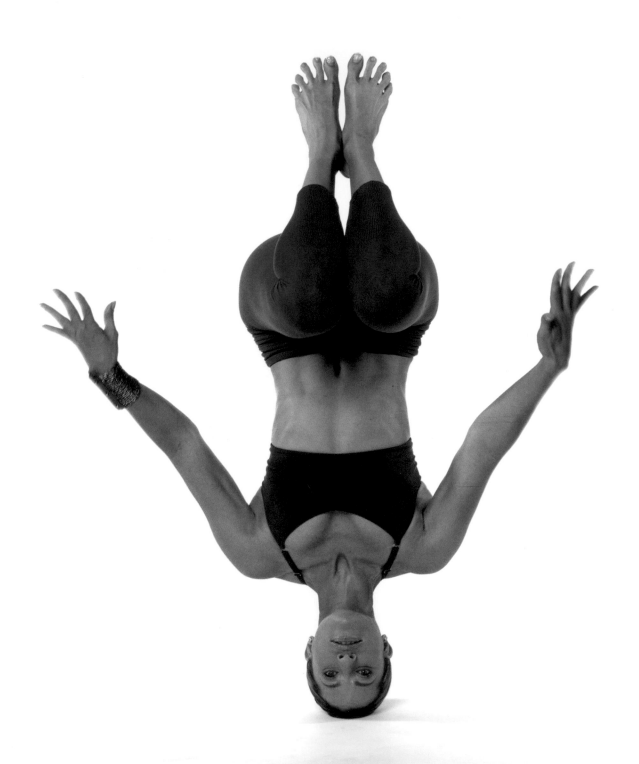

We go forward by going back,

up by going down,

and out by going in.

—RAINBEAU MARS

TODAY IS A
NEW DAY.

CHAPTER 1

BECOMING A SUPERSTAR

Imagine this … You and I are standing together along the bank of a winding, gentle river. It's a beautiful, warm day and we are here to talk about your life—what you want for yourself, who you want to be, and how you want to feel. There is so much you want to do with your life, so much you have to share, and you know that having radiant health and vitality is essential for fulfilling your dreams. But you're not entirely sure how to achieve this state of high health. You've tried different diet and exercise plans. You've invested in the promise of supplements, gym memberships, spa treatments. Yet those things haven't helped you to crack the code of *total* vibrancy. Today is a new day, however, and it is time for you to have all of the energy that you want and need to live your most extraordinary life.

With the moist grass under our feet, we look down at the shimmering water, but it's too enticing to simply observe from the shore! We need to step in and feel the healing current of the waters. With our toes leading the way, we can feel the large river stones welcoming our entrance into the stream of things. But there is an element of trust required just about now, because we can't yet see past the surface to all of the wonders that lie beneath. Muddy waters have been stirred up. The river offers a momentary reflection of what happens within our bodies when the silt and sediment that come from living in our modern world accumulate and circulate within our bodies. The buildup of toxins pollutes the wondrous tributaries within us. The flow of blood and lymph fluid, and the electrical currents of our cellular communication become blocked when we don't give our bodies a cleansing break and a fresh start. But this points to the other part of the story that the river whispers to us today, assuring us that even the murkiest waters can become clear and sparkling again.

Peering into the water once more, we see that the particles of debris are being swept downstream, and the glistening rocks carpeted in lustrous green moss are coming into focus. We can see the fish and underwater flora decorating the bottom of the shallows where we stand. The river murmurs a message that perhaps you've been waiting to hear—one that I believe we all long to hear. It's a reminder that we are a part of the elemental world, a world that is brimming with the resources that can restore us to full functioning—sunlight, air, fruits, vegetables, herbs, and water, to name a few. There is a river of well-being that only requires that we step into it. It is an ever-flowing life force of which we are a part that will sweep away our burdens and support us to fully thrive.

However, there is something required in return. We have to be willing to let the current do its magic—to cleanse us and carry away that which is weighing us down. The system overload can be due to toxins from too many processed foods, energy stagnation from a lack of exercise and fresh air, a pattern of self-neglect carried over from childhood, or any number of factors. Whatever the case may be, we have to be willing to let go of who we are in this moment to become who we *can* be.

Yes, letting go can be hard. We sincerely want change, but then things start to move (the river starts to flow) and we freak out a bit. "Ah, what's going on!?" When we make lifestyle changes that include changes to the way we eat or the way we move our bodies, resistance can surface. Attachments to our familiar comfort foods, resistance to our guides, and other behaviors are entirely understandable and normal. But so many of us equate health, and what it takes to get healthy, with being restrictive. That is a myth I am here to bust once and for all. This program is one where there is no need to panic, because *letting go* in the context of this cleanse program in no way means that you're signing up for a life of austerity and culinary gloom. Hardly! The "gloom" is when we're too exhausted to get excited about life or too sick to really live it. This journey we are embarking upon together is all about shining bright, like your birthright, like you did before you got blocked by fear and doubt. Nature abounds with delicious offerings to delight your palate, restore your physical and emotional exuberance, and rouse your soul.

THE TRUTH IS THAT BECOMING LUMINOUSLY HEALTHY CAN BE A DEEPLY PLEASURABLE EXPERIENCE FOR YOU.

Hundreds of people have thankfully reaped the rewards of *The 21-Day SuperStar Cleanse* as it has evolved over the years, and I become inspired again and again, continuing to share and witness the results, which are a personal renaissance that takes place for the individuals who surrender to this process—*a total renewal of life.*

This program is designed to provide a balance among the following elements:

- Daily guidelines that you can easily customize to fit your needs and goals
- An abundance of irresistible recipes (which are so mouthwatering and easy to make that you just might be inspired to change careers and become a vegan or live foods chef)
- Unwavering support that, if you desire, can extend beyond the pages of this book to include an online community of superstars around the world
- A steady stream of inspiration every day to support you in turning up the dial on your own brilliance

As you envision that amazing light of yours shining more and more brightly, what do you want to do with it? Is there an area of your life where you would like to shine more fully? In your profession? Your intimate relationships? Your parenting? Your creative expression? Your athletic endeavors? Whatever it is that has led you to this program is vitally important, because your superstar glow is needed in this world. And, as the beloved Sufi chant promises, "The ocean refuses no river." It simply awaits your arrival. We will travel together every step of this program, so that you will be provided with clear, practical support as I encourage you to have fun and love yourself through the process.

UNBURDENING THE BODY
the importance of cleansing

Before I outline the program, let's delve a little deeper into how our internal "river" gets so muddy in the first place and how cleansing can quickly turn things around. As the years accumulate, our organs become sluggish from a lifetime of chemical exposure and emotional and environmental toxins, significantly slowing down our metabolism. Even if we live a relatively "clean" and stress-free lifestyle, toxins find a way to intrude. It's hard to escape the air pollution, noise pollution, light pollution, EMFs (electromagnetic frequencies from our cell phones and the other wireless gadgets we love), and even dust mites. The way the body responds to stress, all in a valiant attempt to maintain balance, can result in a less than clean landscape within. Processes and reactions that are meant to be protective *solutions* for handling incoming stress, negative thinking, and toxins—such as inflammation, water retention, and other metabolic and chemical changes—end up becoming part of the *problem*. With the many burdens placed on our bodies over time, there is a decrease in metabolic and digestive enzymes. This can result in our bodies holding on to all kinds of "excess" that weighs us down physically and energetically. Eating nutrient-void foods and overeating them only contributes to excess physical and emotional weight. The real solution, no matter how well we eat, is to *rest, restore,* and *reset.* My favorite teacher, Juan Ruiz, reminded me of a quote: *If you want to know your past, look at your face; your future look at your thoughts.* If we are what we eat, then what we eat also has an effect on what we are thinking, so hand in hand, we can shift who we will be tomorrow by turning over a new leaf today.

Participating in a program like this provides restoration. It nourishes our bodies and minds with a new perspective on food and new ways to approach it, allowing us to release old habits that have contributed to unhealthy, undesirable conditions. Instead of living clouded with toxic residue and putting up with a general state of dis-*ease,* we can reclaim the unbridled enthusiasm that almost every one of us felt as some point in our early lives.

What this means for you is that over these twenty-one days, you can unburden your body and unleash your innate healing and rejuvenating life force. You will be starting from the ground up, rebuilding, restructuring, and refortifying. Without any feelings of restriction, you can reduce (or even eliminate) the input of depleting factors like stress, chemical residues, negative emotions, excess weight, and pollutants on every level. As you nourish your body temple, you will be releasing toxins at the deepest cellular level. As you do this, you will see incredible results in how you feel, how you look, and how you perceive your life.

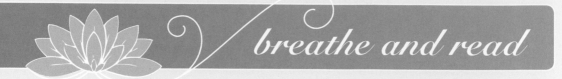

breathe and read

ALIGNING WITH YOUR ULTIMATE POTENTIAL
the key to your success

In the introduction I planted a seed that we will water together throughout the coming three weeks. It is perhaps the single most important aspect of this program. The seed is the absolute knowing that we are here for a purpose, and the tools of this program are designed to support that purpose like never before. The way to sprout that seed and watch it grow is to open to and align with our ultimate potential. These three weeks are designed to support you in completely *embodying* your destiny. Setting an inspiring intention for the three weeks and reclaiming the power of choice will help you to step right into it.

Intention: *Setting Your Intention for the Twenty-One-Day Journey*

What is your primary intention for this process? What would you like to accomplish? It could be a physical outcome, a feeling state, or a shift in perception. It might be very specific or more general and all encompassing. (You can get more specific when it comes time to set your goals.) I would suggest tuning into your future self to set your intention—this is the *you* who has already gone through the cleanse. This future you took a risk to step into the unknown, and you can access that now too. Find that passion for the unknown, for what is fresh. Come to the edge of what it will be like to create something new, and there you will find the intention that is your starting point. In your journal or on a special piece of paper, articulate your intention by completing the following sentence: My superstar cleanse intention is …

Choices: *Making Choices in Alignment with Your Ultimate Potential*

The choices we make every day can serve as either a weapon or a magic wand. The big choices and decisions of life get a lot of attention, but it is the seemingly small ones that might have the biggest impact—like the little bites of food we put into our mouths throughout each day. Recognizing the profound power and impact of choice is the doorway to embodying our highest potential. Each time we prepare to eat something or not, get onto the mat or not, get mired in a limiting belief or emotional state or not, we can ask, "Is this choice in alignment with my highest potential?" Again, you can attune yourself to the future you who has already gone through the cleanse and is feeling wide open, fully nourished, and ready to meet the world. What choices does *that* being make? That is truly the way to embody our ultimate self: let *that* being guide our choices.

Making choices that are in alignment with where we want to be in our deepest being is often met with strong opposition from our egos. The ego rebels, saying, "I'm having that because I *want* it! I'm doing that because I *want* to!" The ego is cozily aligned with what Christian, Buddhist, and other spiritual traditions have called the Seven Deadly Sins. Do you remember learning about those as a kid? Envy, greed, anger, laziness, gluttony, lust, and pride. Because the nature of the ego (a construct of the mind) is built around a perception of separation and isolation, it naturally gravitates toward these energies. They exist in the same resonant field. One concrete example of this is the gluttony we give in to when we eat and drink things that we know are hurting (or even killing) us. So, while the ego is going to go ahead and be its egoic self, the aspect of ourselves that is passionate about waking up can benefit by remembering the *virtues* that counterbalance the sins of the ego, not by stopping the ego from wanting what it wants. There is no bargaining or battling that needs to happen. Instead, we can focus on the benevolent qualities we would like to *add* to our daily lives—and practice things like love, reverence, generosity, dignity, and compassion. With care and attention, these virtuous energies can grow and become stronger. Each day during the cleanse, in the daily Toolkit section, you will find a Virtue of the Day that is provided as a signpost to point the way, to keep you moving in the direction you most want to go. Just as yoga can bring you into anatomical alignment, the virtues can help bring you into alignment at the level of consciousness.

Goals: Setting Your Goals and Committing to Your Ultimate Success

Identifying and clarifying your goals for this journey of transformation will propel you forward over the course of the next twenty-one days, anchoring you to why you have chosen to do this, to what matters most to you right now. If you aren't yet entirely clear about your goals, take some time with your journal or your laptop and make it a fascinating investigation. Ask yourself questions that will help you to sift through your passions and goals: "What's happening in my life right now that needs my attention? Do I have a health issue to address? Do I have weight to lose? If so, how much? Do I have food allergies? What would happen if for the next three weeks I stopped eating wheat and other foods that are most likely making me tired? In what parts of my life would I like to make specific changes? Is there a relationship that I know is keeping me back, but I have not been able to set a boundary? What are the measurable and achievable goals that I most wish to set for this period?" Whether you choose one goal or four, what is most important is that your goals motivate you to reach, stretch, and expand without being overwhelming. If there is a second tier of goals, consider saving those for your next time around with this program. (You can use it to stoke the fires of your superstar self for years to come.)

As you are clarifying your goals, ask yourself, "Is this goal in alignment with my ultimate potential?" Any goal that calls you into alignment, that propels you to live that potential more and more, is worth your energy and attention.

You might have a goal to lose ten pounds, or to wake up in the morning feeling rested and totally alive, or to have the energy in the evenings to spend quality time with your partner, hobby, or children. You might also have a goal to run a marathon, to get in shape for the new public speaking career you're going after, to revive your sex life, or to attract a worthy relationship in the first place. You can have several goals, and no matter how large or small, they can all be in service to your ultimate purpose. After all, your ultimate purpose is something to be lived *each* day, not a destination to be reached one day down the road.

Here's the thing about goals: To achieve them, we usually have to let something go, at least for a while. (Yes, it's the "letting go" challenge again.) But we must be strong! To get the most out of this cleanse, we need to step away from a few habits that are deleterious to our health. Breaking up is hard to do but so worthwhile, when necessary. It's like that boyfriend or girlfriend you know is bad for you, but you keep calling them back, even though each time you partake you feel sick. They're just so addicting, right? Well, we can't change them, but we can change ourselves, and we can replace the old habits with good ones and be free from addiction. Week One is the time we say good-bye to any old toxic relationships to anything or anyone that's not serving us. And who doesn't slip with a phone call or two just to be sure? Same goes with steering into the drive-through fast-food restaurant. I am here to firmly remind you that you have made your intentions clear and set your goals, so for the sake of your integrity, please keep on driving, walking, and forgivingly putting the phone down. By Week Two you will be saying hello to your new and improved life with room for what's fresh. With the abundance of mineral-rich, high-water-content, healing superfoods, you'll hardly miss your old diet. During Week Three, you will be taking your life to the next level by possibly indulging in more bioavailable blended foods and juices, further boosting your metabolism for renewed energy and beauty. With a little added structure and healthy discipline, you will be resetting your entire system and discovering how quickly your body gives back to you. After the three-week cleanse, you will find that "the old toxic relationship" no longer holds the same allure. You will be far more captivated by the energetic shift that is taking place, where you are feeling new sensations, thinking new thoughts, and watching in amazement as some of the things you've wanted to attract start coming to you with greater ease. I frequently observe with my friends and clients how they magnetize possibilities and opportunities by changing their vibration through cleansing. As we *open, align*, and *reset*, we draw in jobs, money, relationships, collaborative opportunities, inner states of peace and joy, or whatever is in our heart to attract.

Prepare to be your own personal growth coach, saying to yourself, "For three weeks I'm going to follow the plan and do everything that supports my well-being. I'm going to try new recipes, move my body, and read things that stimulate my creativity and intelligence. I'm going to play, listen to new music, journal, and more. Afterward, we'll focus on integrating and reentering our lives with a healthy new perspective.

It's important to begin this journey fully acknowledging that egos will assert themselves at times, seemingly hijacking us into failure. You might give in during the three-week cleanse period. But don't judge yourself if this happens! Cravings or reasons to make you feel you can't do this will come up. But in the areas of life where you have found success, have there not also been challenges? Drama may approach, people's words of doubt may get to you, or perhaps you'll forget to pack food before a long day out. I invite you to simply pick up from there; you can't lose, only gain more insight. "So I had some coffee, or some bread. I will choose to observe myself and plan out what I can do next time the trigger arises. I don't have to go back to square one." Perfection isn't the purpose or goal of this process. It's about something far more beautiful. It's the gradual experience of waking up.

Are you ready to commit to doing what it takes? I find that breaking the one big commitment down into nine bite-sized commitments is a way to set ourselves up to win. In preparation for this journey, you will read the nine commitments on the next page and revisit them throughout this cleanse. If you wish to read through a bit more of the program to know what to expect, then okay. But please come back to this page and read the commitments out loud when you are ready.

Okay, so now it's time. Let's raise our right hands together and say the commitments out loud and proud. Do you want to increase the power of your commitment? Say them out loud to a mirror, a video camera, or a friend. Say each one twice, please, to really hear the words you are saying. And it all begins with the word … and so it is.

ATTENTION, PLEASE! Each time you embark on *The 21-Day SuperStar Cleanse* process, I recommend that you renew your commitments. One of the strongest ways to do this is to post the commitments in a place where you can see them often during the three weeks, such as in your bedroom, bathroom, or kitchen. Also, signing your name and writing down the date is powerful reinforcement. Therefore, I have made a printable version of the Nine Commitments available at: 21daysuperstarcleanse.com. Go there now to access your free, downloadable PDF.

THE NINE COMMITMENTS
for achieving your superstar glow

1. I am committed to following this program to the very best of my ability.
2. I am committed to nourishing myself with foods of the highest quality.
3. I am committed to decreasing and preferably avoiding addictive substances for the next twenty-one days. I know that to be my most clear self, I must release addictive patterns and intoxicants including drugs, alcohol, cigarettes, harmful foods, and toxic relationships.
4. I am committed to avoiding chemical substances—including toxins found in foods, cleaning products, beauty products, and other environmental hazards—and investigating alternatives.
5. I am committed to seeing this journey as a growth process where love, harmony, acceptance, and compassion reign supreme. Therefore, I relinquish any need, desire, or impulse to judge others, this process, or myself.
6. I am committed to listening to, loving, and living fully in my body during this time. This includes giving myself at least thirty minutes of daily exercise or meditation such as walking, Qigong, dance, yoga, surfing, Pilates, Tantric breathing in an upward direction, and/or positive visualization.
7. I am committed to forgiving others and myself on a daily basis. Forgiveness is a vital practice for succeeding with this program and living a healthy, happy life.
8. I am committed to listening to the inner voice of my being, not my ego, at all times during the next twenty-one days. I promise to trust my intuition and know that the guidance system of my heart will always choose the most healing path for aligning with my ultimate purpose and my best self.
9. I am committed to being Love, and I will strengthen this commitment by being in integrity with my thoughts, words, and actions.

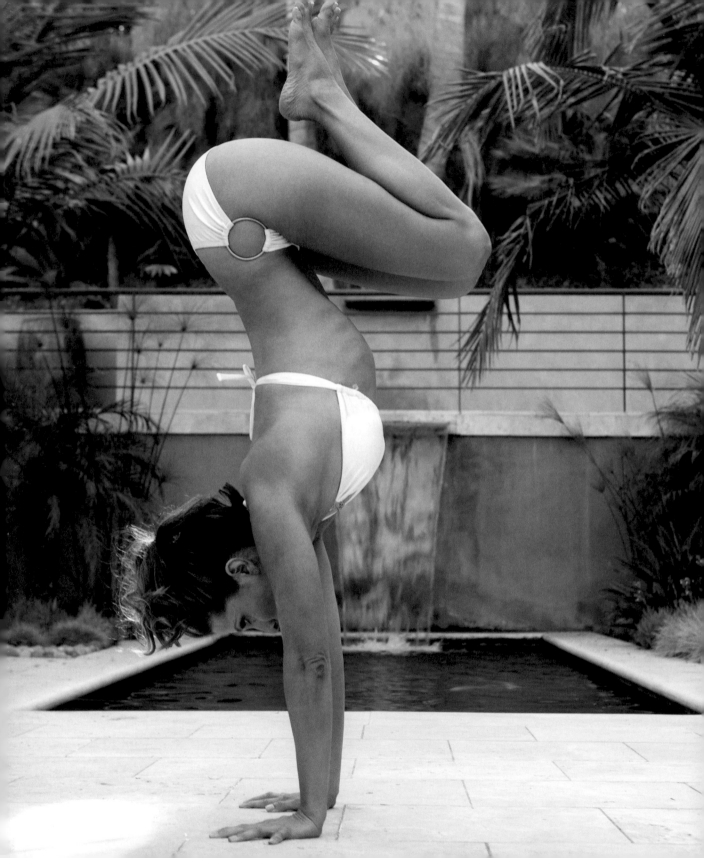

Your overall commitment to the twenty-one-day program will keep you in action toward your goals. In this context, your commitment is the promise you make to yourself to put self-love into action and fully engage in the process.

PHYSICAL TRANSFORMATIONS
WHAT TO EXPECT

- Radiant, glowing skin
- A reduction of fine lines and wrinkles
- Increased energy
- Deeper, more restful sleep
- Decreased amount of time needed to sleep, while feeling completely rested
- Weight stabilization—your body can become its ideal weight
- Reduction of cellulite and other skin-related issues such as acne or eczema
- Alleviation of mood swings and overall improved mood
- Unraveling of physical knots and tension in the body
- Greater flexibility and stamina
- Increased attention span and a better ability to focus
- Improved memory
- Mental clarity, increased creativity, and inspiration
- Feeling "high" and happy without the use of stimulants or substances of any kind

PREPARATIONS FOR YOUR TWENTY-ONE-DAY JOURNEY
your structures for success

From setting up your pantry and stocking your fridge to asking your community of loved ones for their support and scheduling time for yourself in your calendar, there are a few simple but crucial steps to take in preparation for your twenty-one-day program. In addition to the core intention, choices, goals, and commitments you have now begun to contemplate, the information to follow will completely round out the inner and outer structures for your success.

Embracing Your Kitchen

There are certain appliances, superfoods, supplements, and kitchen preparations that I have found especially helpful for the twenty-one-day program. However, before you get acquainted with them, please note that this is not a must-have checklist. Since you may choose to use this program in the future (such as seasonally and prior to important milestone moments in your life), I recommend that you gradually incorporate a few of these suggestions each time or at a pace that fits comfortably with your budget.

HIGH-QUALITY BLENDER
Vitamix blenders are highly recommended, though there are many quality high-speed blenders on the market. Even if you don't intend to remain 100 percent vegan or raw after the cleanse, it is truly one of the best investments you can make.

DEHYDRATOR
Live-foodists tend to prefer the Excalibur brand of dehydrator. A solar oven will work as well, and if you're somewhere really hot, you can just use a screen to keep the bugs away. If this is not an option for you, you can also try cracking your oven door open while it's on a low, warm setting. Just do the best you can and explore. There are many options for "uncooking" with the appliances you have in your kitchen (think toaster ovens, window sills, and more).

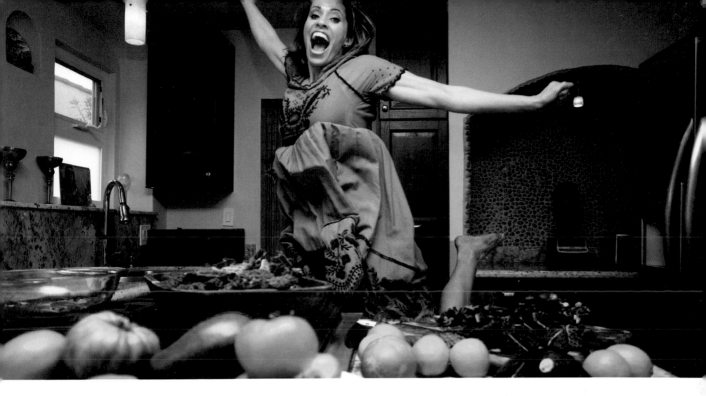

FOOD PROCESSOR

A food processor is an excellent tool for any kitchen. It helps when chopping nuts or making thick purees and doughs. It can even serve as a substitute blender. Waring and Cuisinart produce good ones.

KITCHEN UTENSILS

Make sure you have a great strainer, a cutting board, and high-quality sharp knives.

JUICER

Juicing vegetables, herbs, and fruits is an exceptional way to condense the nutrients of these foods into potent, enzyme-rich drinks. There are several excellent juicers on the market, from the Breville to the Greenstar and beyond.

CITRUS JUICER

These little beauties are cheap (as little as $3), efficient, and useful beyond measure. One of the great beauty enhancers internally and externally, lemon juice is a vital aspect of this program, given its alkalizing effect on the body. So your citrus juicer will be put to good use.

SUPERFOODS

We now live in a world of superfood abundance, which is good news because superfoods equal beauty foods! Superfoods are plant-based foods containing high amounts of antioxidants and phytochemicals, which are protective, disease-preventing compounds. These nutrient-dense foods go a step beyond our luscious, organically grown fruits and vegetables, offering a powerful concentration of vitamins, minerals, and other micronutrients. Now available everywhere (especially when you consider the Internet), they are a vital component for anyone looking to achieve and sustain a superstar glow. While I also list them in the weekly shopping list sections for the three weeks of the cleanse, in brief I would like to highlight and recommend the following superfoods: maca, acai, cacao, lucuma, camu camu, goji berries, noni juice, tocotrienols (a potent form of vitamin E), chia seeds, and durian (a large tropical fruit revered in Southeast Asian countries, nutrient rich and possessing a distinct aroma!). Explore what you like and tune in to what your body responds to and requires to function optimally. *Note: You will find descriptions of most of these superfoods in the Week One Recommended Shopping List section on pages 85 to 89.*

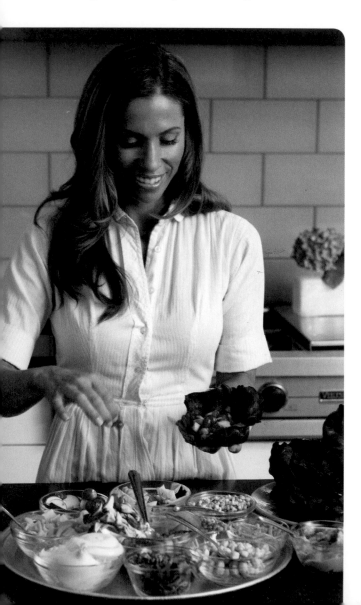

DIGESTIVE ENZYMES

Digestive enzymes break down proteins, fats, carbohydrates, and fiber, supporting our ability to utilize the nutrients we ingest. In essence, they turn the foods we eat into energy. Buy a good digestive enzyme supplement and take a few each time you eat cooked foods (primarily during Week One of the cleanse). My favorite brands are Ascended Health and Premier Research Labs. *Note: For more information on enzymes, see "Enzymes in Living Foods" on pages 201 to 202 and "More Reasons to Eat Enzymes" on page 203.*

DELIVERY OPTIONS

Look into delivery options from your local vegan or live food restaurants or ready-made to-go options at your local health food store. You may even consider partnering with an individual or community support group that switches off the duties of chef, giving you some free days. This will of course also help expand your health team, which is important for your long-term goals of success.

SWITCH TO GLASS OR CERAMICS

Plastic leaches chemicals into whatever it touches—bottled water, juices, packaged and wrapped foods, body care products, and other items. Invest in quality glass storage containers and pitchers to eliminate the unnecessary toxins that can disrupt your endocrine system and hormones, contributing to weight gain and a host of other health and environmental issues.

PREPARE AHEAD

Prepare your menu in advance. Shop and prepare snacks to have on hand so that you are not tempted to make questionable last-minute food choices when you feel like you're starving or your blood sugar drops. By preparing in advance, you will also save money when you order items in bulk or shop from a raw food wholesale club. Please take the time to go to a farmer's market, health food store, or co-op near you. While supporting your local farmers, you will also be ensuring that you are getting the freshest and most vital produce possible. Always buy what looks healthy, bright, delicious, and fun. Remember: you are what you eat.

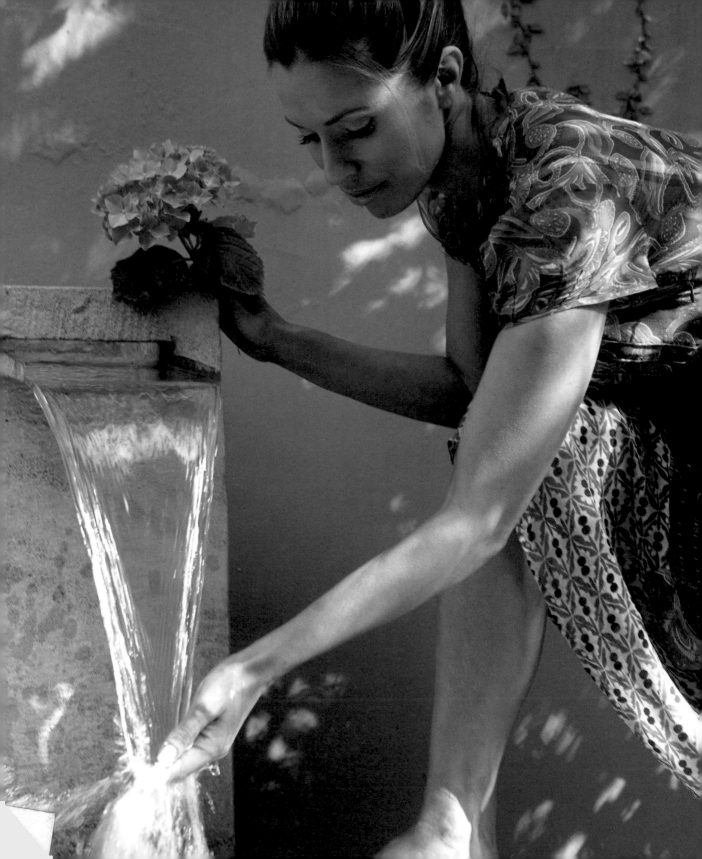

Creating a Sanctuary for Transformation

CHOOSING YOUR SANCTUARY

When we are undergoing change that involves an excavation of some of the thoughts, feelings, beliefs, and perceptions that we have held deeply within ourselves, we need to create a sacred space where we are free and safe to explore this internal landscape. If at all possible, designate a space within your home that serves this purpose, whether that is a room, a corner, a closet, or an altar. If this is not ideal, find a place in nature or a favorite public place where you can reflect, connect, and honor your process.

ABOUT CLEANING YOUR SANCTUARY

We will go into this in greater depth later, but I need to remind you that it's best if your sanctuary is as clean as possible, with as few environmental hazards as possible. Consider an air filter and clean it as you would a temple area that has been loved up and cleaned out with nontoxic environmental products.

MAKING TIME FOR YOUR SANCTUARY

Your sanctuary is a place where you can observe yourself and not be distracted by toxicity on any level. Set aside a time when you can be peaceful within your environment of choice. If you are someone whose schedule is filled to capacity most days, give yourself at least five minutes a day (with the intent of gently expanding this time allotment as your capacity for self-care increases). Make this your favorite time of day at a place and time that make you feel peaceful and happy. This is a harmonious time in which you can rest, journal, read inspirational books, exercise, listen to self-help audios, watch life-affirming DVDs, or engage in anything that makes you feel divine. Take healing baths, go to the spa, get a massage, or take a yoga class. Gift yourself with anything you know will support your transformation. These twenty-one days are an opportunity to shift your attention from being outwardly focused to aligning within.

Toxins don't only come from pollution in the environment: stress has 82,000 contraindications, so make peace in your life and in all relations. Since you are embarking on a journey of detoxification, do your best to refrain from interactions with less than supportive places or things, including people, at this time. Go ahead and welcome insights like "know thyself," as this is truly what this experience is about. It's a turning inward to know thy healthier and more authentic self. Please vow to remain conscious and kind to yourself and others, which at times will involve sturdier boundaries.

Surrounding Yourself with Love and Support

This is the time to realize and visualize who you really are. Every step you take during this process needs to support your intention. You might want to invite in one or two honest, loving, and compassionate people whom you can call on when you are tempted to fall into old patterns. Choose wisely, as you will need to be sure they will offer their support, and most important, they will continue to root for you even if you struggle at times. This may be a close friend to either join you on this program or simply be a supportive presence for you while you're on your clearing journey. This may also be a teacher, mentor, or life coach. These days, there are many different kinds of support groups; for instance, we have an online forum you can join. If others in your home are not joining you on giving up addictive foods, kindly ask that they still support *your* decision by either refraining from comment or offering words of encouragement and helping you resist temptation if you need it.

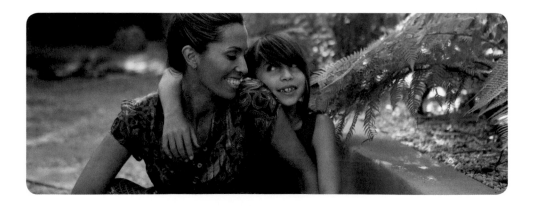

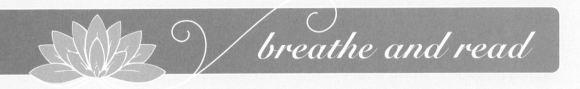

breathe and read

THE TOOLS OF TRANSFORMATION
getting to know your superstar cleanse blueprint

For ease of use, each week of the cleanse has been assigned its own color-coding so you can quickly reference the pages that are most important to you along the way. To guide you elegantly through each day and week of the program, the following chapter components provide the blueprint for an experience that will be both pleasurable and effective:

CUSTOMIZING YOUR SUPERSTAR PLAN
Food and diet suggestions for beginner, intermediate, and advanced cleansers. Reading about each option will help you decide where you are comfortable, finding the balance between challenging yourself and being gentle with yourself.

PREPARING FOR YOUR SUPERSTAR GLOW
Easy and enjoyable assignments (aka "homework") suggested for preparing for the week as a whole.

RECOMMENDED SHOPPING LIST
Suggested foods, condiments, and supplements for preparing the meals that will restore or increase your inner and outer glow.

YOUR DAILY SCHEDULE
Each day of the three weeks begins with an overview of the day—suggested meals, tonics, juices, and activities that you can adapt to meet your needs. From dawn to dusk, you can use this as your touchstone for staying on track. When you are in the integration part and contemplation part of the work after

the cleanse, you will have an opportunity to mix and match your favorite meal choices and practices to suit your needs as you begin to make your re-entry into a new healthy routine.

Note: As you will see, the recommended time for dinner during the three weeks of the cleanse is 6:00 p.m., which can further support a break for your digestive system. If your schedule allows you to eat dinner even earlier, that's great. However, these are only suggestions. If you need to eat later, that's fine as well, but opt to have your breakfast later than the suggested 8:00 a.m. time frame as well, to provide an ample overnight fast.

YOUR DAILY TOOLKIT

The Toolkit section is the anchor for each day of the three-week cleanse. In it you will find the following tools for enlightening your body and uplifting your consciousness:

- **Virtue of the Day:** Inspiration for an empowered mindset.
- **Action Step of the Day:** Activities to support your alignment with your ultimate potential.
- **Recipe of the Day:** Enjoy this specially selected meal recipe or choose another from Rainbeau's Recipe Roundup section on page 304.
- **Yoga Pose of the Day:** Feel your best by moving your body! The style of yoga on this cleanse will be either classic *Yoga for Beauty* or *ra'yoKa*, the seven-level system that I developed. For an introduction to *ra'yoKa*, see pages 61 to 69.
- **Mantra of the Day:** Your focusing tool for superstar success.

ILLUMINATIONS

Supplemental information pertaining to the specific week of the cleanse process to increase your knowledge base and fire up your motivation. Grab a cup of caffeine-free chai or a fresh juice and further expand your mind.

REFLECTIONS

Inspiration for journaling and self-inquiry.

In addition to the daily and weekly blueprint provided in chapters 1 through 5, I have created two special sections that you will refer to throughout the twenty-one days (and can also use as resources in your healthy future).

RAINBEAU'S RECIPE ROUNDUP

Starting on page 304, you will find my comprehensive superstar collection of recipes. This includes each recipe suggested throughout the cleanse, as well as bonus recipes that you can use interchangeably, depending on what appeals to you. In addition to the detailed recipes, this section also includes a recipe index:

- Your quick-reference guide for finding recipes by name or by type (entrées, soups, salads, snacks, vegan breakfasts, desserts, shakes, smoothies, juices, and tonics)

RAINBEAU'S READING ROOM

Starting on page 343, you will find the doorway to a wealth of supplemental information for further enriching and fortifying your experience. You know the saying …

KNOWLEDGE IS POWER

Equipped with these support structures and guidelines, the coming twenty-one days will surpass your wildest expectation if you are willing to do the following:

PRIORITIZE YOURSELF

Put yourself on the top of your list daily. Contrary to being selfish, this will only enable you to give more to everyone else around you. What you feed yourself, both physically (food) and emotionally (thoughts), represents how you feel about yourself. By changing just one of these, you can shift the other. As you change your diet to delicious, nourishing, and healing choices, you can watch your thoughts take on a more positive outlook. Shift your thoughts to those of love, self-worth, and confidence, and watch how you will be naturally and magnetically drawn to the foods that will nurture, energize, and support your body. As I will remind you throughout, self-care is a major component of this program. If this is difficult for you (as it is for many people), I invite you to use your quiet times to compassionately investigate and journal about any resistance or beliefs you encounter concerning what it means to take care of yourself.

EXPRESS YOURSELF

Invest in a designated new journal or art book for the program. Write, draw, collage, or paint pictures in it that allow you to deeply express yourself through the process. You can also visualize or even sing about your experience, giving voice to what you crave, miss, need, and hope for. I believe that what is most important about journaling and other forms of self-expression is that they give us a way to be close and intimate with ourselves throughout any process like this cleanse—like a dear friend who is listening, witnessing, and simply being present with the truth of the moment. The more we embrace ourselves without judgment, the more we can move onward with acceptance. Then we can breathe into a *new* space that we didn't realize we had, like moving into a new house—only this house is our dream house.

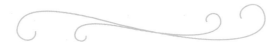

DISCOVERING RA'YOKA
yoga for sports and yoga for beauty

Throughout the twenty-one-day program, you will have the opportunity to explore *ra'yoKa*, the seven-level system of practice developed to harmonize body, mind, and life. Each day of the three weeks of the cleanse program, I will guide you through a pose to introduce you to the benefits of yoga or *ra'yoKa* at a gentle yet steady pace. By the end, when you move into the culminating period of the program, you will have familiarity with this unique practice and can choose to incorporate the poses that give you the results you want. For the more classical static poses, we use the term *Yoga for Beauty* from two of my programs. For an in-depth, dynamic series of sequencing, you'll want to order some downloads or DVDs from www.rainbeaumarslifestyles.com. There is even a virtual teacher training available there for a thorough life-enriching study that includes Skype time with me.

So, what is ra'yoKa?

The *ra'yoKa* system combines the fundamental principles of classical yoga, enhanced with a breath-centered flow, dynamic and explosive martial arts movements, and an emphasis on one's core connection. It is a total body balance integration system that merges physical, mental, and spiritual elements with the intention of awakening the mind and body.

While maintaining and respecting the roots of the Ashtanga yoga laws of nonharm (*ahisma*) and truth (*satya*), as well as the niyamas (personal ethics) and yamas (social ethics) that are the first two limbs of yoga's eight-fold path, *it veers out into a riskier realm of incorporating the present-day need for hybridizing explosive power-giving movement.* The name *ra'yoKa* comes from the Sanskrit root word "ra," representing the sun, and the word "yoka," which evolved from the word "yoga"— meaning "to yoke," to integrate and unify the mind and body.

Integration of the Sun Through the Nadis: Ida, Pingala, and Sushumna

The focus and intention of *ra'yoKa* is the integration and embodiment of the sun—in all its dynamic aliveness. The illuminating star at the center of our solar system mirrors our own center, or solar plexus, and the 72,000 channels of light (*nadis* in Sanskrit) that run through it. The three main *nadis*—*ida* (the feminine aspect of receiving), *pingala* (the masculine aspect of giving), and *sushumna* (the merging of all that invites balance and transcendence)—are honored and nourished through the practice of *ra'yoKa*—as well as through each week of the twenty-one-day cleanse. In *ra'yoKa*, like a sun ray that is housed through the center of the spine, we draw *sushumna* to the center. Physiologically, when *sushumna* is activated through the opening of the spine, it also saturates and awakens the brain hemispheres with endorphins and melatonin.

Yoga, ra'yoKa, and You

The hybrid *ra'yoKa* system is intended to bring you into anatomical alignment, where your body as a whole teaches your brain what alignment *feels* like. I know that when I get on the mat and do my practice, I see and feel my ultimate potential. I continue to evolve *ra'yoKa* in order to embody and know my whole self. That is my desire for you too as you journey through the twenty-one days of this program. As you explore the daily poses, breathing *sushumna* to and through your solar plexus (the merging of the 72,000 *nadis* of subtle energy and light), my dream is that the ray of light that you are shines more brightly than ever before, for you and for all those you come across. My hope is that you can be an ignited torch and pass this on to others.

RA'YOKA COLOR CHART

LEVELS OF CONTENT	BODY LOCATION	ELEMENTS & THEMES	PHYSICAL FOCUS
Level Violet: *Meditation*	Crown	Union: *Consciousness*	Recalibration through mediation, affirmation & openness
Level Indigo: *Inversions*	Upper Brow	Visualization: *Balance, Insight*	Mental focus, balance, breath, inversions, visualization & intentions
Level Blue: *Therapeutics*	Throat	Sound: *Communication, Clarity*	Vocal & body harmony through mantras, sound, throat & jaw openers
Level Green: *Backbends*	Chest	Air: *Opening, Gratitude*	Heart & chest openers, shoulder openers & back bends, with breathing exercises
Level Yellow: *Core Power*	Solar Plexus	Fire: *Power*	Core strength & fluidity, with side stretches, core lifting, arm balances, core crunches & twists
Level Orange: *Detoxification*	Pelvic Floor	Water: *Creativity*	Twists, uddiyana bandhas, groin, reproductive, & sexual meridians, digestion & elimination support
Level Red: *Foundation*	Legs	Earth: *Material*	Standing poses, focus on cardiovascular, alignment, gross movement, legs, hips openers, ankles & feet

ELEMENTS OF RA'YOKA
the flowering of influences

Benefits of ra'yoKa

THE PSYCHOLOGICAL BENEFITS OF RA'YOKA THROUGH FOCUS

The therapeutic benefits of meditation, breath, movement, and visualization allow you to disconnect from day-to-day stress while relieving tension and anxiety.

- Provides mental clarity and concentration through deliberate intention of practice
- Promotes a sense of strength, empowerment, and confidence

THE PHYSICAL BENEFITS OF RA'YOKA THROUGH MOVEMENT

- Stimulates fast-and-slow twitch muscles, which increases power and reactive abilities
- Deliberately draws attention toward focus on the practice, developing commitment and self-discipline
- Strengthens the musculoskeletal structure through balance, dynamic lunges, twists, and core stabilizing, while increasing power with explosive movements
- Builds and releases energy
- Improves core strength, stability, balance, coordination, and agility
- Prevents injuries through understanding proper alignment and correct technique

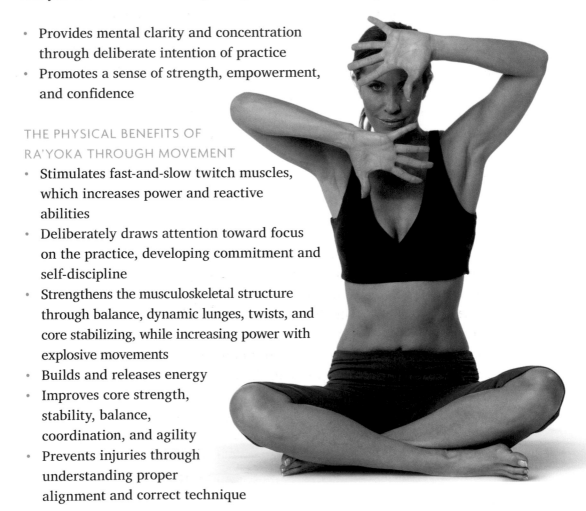

- Balances hormones and emotions
- Demonstrates proper breathing during practice, increasing the amount of oxygen available to the body
- Improves flexibility and mobility, increasing range of motion
- Helps ease pain and relieves muscle tension
- Helps to improve body alignment through body and spatial awareness
- Aids weight control efforts by regulating metabolism, reducing the cortisol levels, burning excess calories, and reducing stress
- Helps improve circulation, nourishing organs with fresh, oxygenated blood through the detoxifying poses such as twists
- Provides cardiovascular benefits by lowering resting heart rate, increasing endurance, and improving oxygen uptake during exercise
- Promotes reaction to challenging moments with a nonreactionary mind
- Improves reaction time, memory, and focus

THE SPIRITUAL BENEFITS OF RA'YOKA THROUGH BREATHING

- Helps bring attention to the present, eliminating negative thoughts and improving mind and body awareness
- Identifies intentions: strong like fire, calm like air, or soothing like water
- Combines emotional intention with the breath and physical practice to enhance the whole body experience (example: "I open when I inhale, and I get stronger when I exhale")
- Clears out and liberates the chakras, or inner energy centers of our bodies, with visualization, breath, and movement
- Recognizes and balances our *inner bodies*, our emotional and mental patterns that have an effect on the rest of our being
- The foundation of the practice stems from the expansion and contraction of the core, elongating the muscles, finding length with each inhale, contracting and integrating with the exhale to prevent injuries and hyperextension. We match each breath to movement so we remember to maintain free movement internally (keeping oxygen in the muscles and the mind as relaxed as possible), eliminating unnecessary tension

Benefits of Yoga and ra'yoKa Body Positions

SEATED

Calming positions that refresh both brain and body, helping remove fatigue and calm stressed nerves. These poses fall into two categories: upright postures and forward bends.

STANDING

Invigorating positions that teach a blueprint of alignment for every posture. They are like coming home, remembering your intention, or coming back to zero. Standing correctly is an important tool in aligning one's body and patterns of the mind.

STANDING POSES

Develop awareness of correct body alignment for sitting, standing, and walking. These are fantastic hip aligners and create a strong foundation for the rest of the body. They are the support system. The quadriceps are the largest muscles in the body and can create heat and warmth through the whole system.

QUICK KICKS OR PUNCHES

Work the fast-twitch muscles and the ability to move quickly and powerfully. They create a cardiovascular kickstart that builds heat. They promote confidence, quick thinking, agility, and an overall body intelligence that creates power.

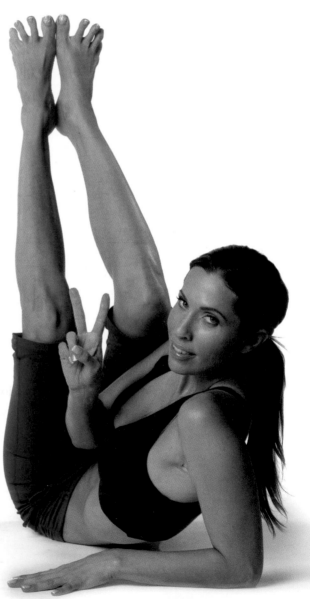

TWISTS

Excellent for detoxification and massaging of the internal organs, releasing tension, and promoting increased blood flow and circulation throughout the entire body. Great for spinal release, overall fluidity, and body movement.

BALANCE POSTURES, STATIC AND NONSTATIC

Develop control over the body and stabilize major joint-system and balance muscles. Improve coordination, concentration, focus, and the overall ability to stay centered in the midst of chaos. Discover how to be both strong and grounded while simultaneously fluid and relaxed.

SUPINE AND PRONE

Promote improved mobility and stability of the torso and hips. Certain ones strengthen the upper body and others relax the body. They change one's perspective and move the mind into a more receptive, subconscious state, which is beneficial for transformation.

BACK BENDS

The heart of the practice … literally. Back bends promote circulation, digestion, and complete restructuring of the overall body, especially the spine. Good for the nervous and glandular systems, promoting endorphin release and stimulating expanded awareness. When practiced correctly, they can heal the body from a multitude of disorders, including back pain, depression, heartache, anxiety, osteoporosis, and longevity … for we are as young as our back is mobile.

FORWARD BENDS

Forward bends are essential for elongating the spine and maintaining the soft tissue between the vertebrae. They are recommended for mild detoxification, hamstring release, and leg lengthening, and are beneficial in opening of the hips and counterposing back bends.

INVERTED

Considered the king and queen of yoga postures. Reverse gravity and support the endocrine and nervous systems. Revitalize the body and improve circulation. Inverted poses support concentration, digestion, and sleep, and promote relaxation and tranquility. Also great for detoxification.

HIP OPENERS

The hip joint is the largest joint in the body, home to the garbage pail of old emotional and chemical toxins. It can be flushed and cleansed by spending time relaxing, breathing, and affirming healing that focuses on the area. Be aware that opening the body and often the hips can result in emotional releases.

EYE AND JAW EXERCISES

Both of these can subtly, yet precisely, balance the brain hemispheres and release habitual patterning of the face (including wrinkles). They can free the nervous system, improve concentration and focus, and increase the brain's ability to think efficiently, creatively, and clearly.

MEDITATION

Promotes pointed concentration, clear thinking, and manifestation abilities. It is the pause and clarity in the midst of being, a chance to observe and listen.

VISUALIZATION

Whatever we focus on expands. Rather than focusing on "the impossible," we can intentionally use visualization to see the chakras aligned and infused with new energy and light. We can envision oxygen rejuvenating the cells and healing every corner of the body.

CHANTING AFFIRMATIONS

Support the overall harmony of the energies of the cellular, emotional, and anatomical structure. Create resonance and clarity in the entire physical instrument. We can only think of one thing at a time, so if our brain is being used to affirm positive things, any negative thought patterning falls away.

RESTORATIVES/SAVASANA

It is very important to "get out of the way" on a regular basis and allow gravity to align the bones and draw us open into a more relaxed and supported state. Restoratives are excellent after traveling contraindications. To be used for digestion, menstrual and prenatal symptoms, serious sickness, or even to restore the physical/mental/emotional bodies after or during trauma.

PRANAYAMA

The yogis say that "controlled breathing" should be practiced when there is already a general mastery of the body. It is dangerous to hold the breath, but can be very beneficial for a multitude of disorders and can enhance the positive qualities of a practice by at least double. Recommended for calming the mind and nervous systems, increasing one's meditative state, and mastering one-pointed concentration.

Recently, I have been pondering the metaphor of parachuting. I'm sure this is because I've been making many big changes and stepping into new, exciting, and unfamiliar territory. You know that feeling when you're stepping out onto the edge of your known world. I think many of us know that we are ready. It is time to try it—it's time to make the jump into new levels of health, into a new experience of life. We want the thrill *and* the dramatic internal shift that will follow as a result of our act of courage.

Yet we want to stay planted in our seat on the plane too, holding onto what we have known, only jumping if we are guaranteed that upon landing we will still be the person we have known. Flirting with the idea of never forgoing our comfort zone, we cling to the past.

Today, we need not carry the extra burdens and baggage of all we have known. My challenge for you, me, and everyone else reading these words is this: LET'S JUMP! The parachutes are here! Let's hold hands and breathe: 1 … 2 … 3 … Freedom and health are waiting. Yes, it's time. Let us look directly at our excuses, attachments, patterns, and fears and kindly ask them to please step aside. Let's jump and let's transform without looking back.

Are you in? As in … with me? I hope so …

LET'S DO THIS!

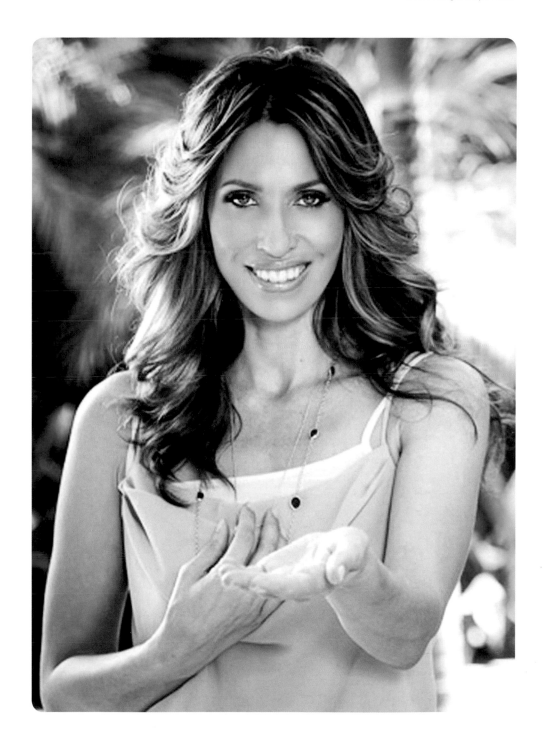

NOW ALL WE HAVE
TO DO IS BEGIN ...
LET'S LET OUR TRUE,
BEAUTIFUL SELVES
BE OUR OFFERING.

CHAPTER 2

WEEK ONE: REBALANCING WITH THE VEGAN DIET

One of my most memorable clients is Nicolas, a successful business manager in his fifties who embarked on *The 21-Day SuperStar Cleanse* program never having heard of eating all vegan much less live foods. Eating a plant-based diet free of all animal-derived products (including dairy and eggs) simply had never occurred to him. Nicolas works with tremendous drive and enthusiasm, and like many of us, loves to reward himself with great meals, treats, and snacks. Over the years he had become a well-known patron of some of the best sushi restaurants and other high-end hangouts in Los Angeles, including wine clubs. Despite the good life he had created for himself, when Nicolas first started the program he had a hard time breathing deeply, slept with breathing strips over his nose, had constant, chronic coughs, and was on a high level of cholesterol medicine. He knew he could feel much better than he did, but didn't realize it would start from within and with what he was consuming. Nicolas started the program at the beginner's level (which you will learn about shortly) and eased his way into a new way of eating, which meant incorporating meat substitutes and other comfort foods like tempeh, rice and beans, ample sweet potatoes, and lots of soups. He was a great sport about trying new things and was amazed to discover that he could feel completely satisfied without fish, meat, or dairy. He would also be the first to admit that the feedback he began to receive from the people around him fanned the flames of his excitement to complete the program. As they noticed his rosy cheeks and the warm light emanating from his eyes, friends started cheering him on. He had more fun than he expected to through the various phases of the cleanse, which had him making up some of his own motivational mantras, such as, "I can't wait for tomorrow, because I get better looking every day!"

The internal changes were at least as thrilling as the external benefits. By the end of the program, Nicolas had lost twenty-two pounds, had his cholesterol medicine nearly cancelled, and heard from his doctor that his blood test was the best it had ever been.

Nicolas's health and energy are consistently strong now, not only because of the few twenty-one-day cleanses themselves but also because of the quality of the choices he continues to make each day. And because he isn't carrying around low-level anxiety about his heart health any longer, he is more relaxed and confident. His extra energy is being used for winning golf tournaments and pursuing new interests. Fueled by his newfound love of chia seed porridge for breakfast and kale salads at any time of the day, Nicolas said, "Go ahead and share my story, because if I can enjoy eating vegan, then anyone can!"

Now it's your turn to heal and transform. For the entirety of this twenty-one-day program, you are invited to indulge in all things living and vegan. The great revelation for those who try a vegan diet, either as part of the program or even on a long-term basis, is the discovery that food really can be *both* delicious and healthy. This is your opportunity to experience the best of both worlds while reaping the mental and physical benefits of a plant-based diet.

While I invite you to experiment with plant-based and living food recipes as well as the many vegan products at your natural foods grocery store, I remind you to avoid the vegan junk food. This program encourages whole foods—often directly from the garden—not processed, fried, or white sugar or gluten filled that can be common in an unhealthy vegan food diet.

Our focus together is on exploring all those vegetables, exotic fruits, healthy fats, whole grains, and seeds you may never have tried or known how to prepare in a delicious way. The mainstay of any diet should always be plant-based foods, as that is where we get our minerals, vitamins, antioxidants, fiber, and enzymes.

I want to encourage you to indulge. Eat and try foods without thinking about amounts, as long as you stick to the parameters. There is absolutely no deprivation on this program. Following our guidelines doesn't mean that there aren't ample opportunities to have your cake and eat it too; on the contrary, that's what it's all about. In fact, there are many ways to indulge on this program and never feel guilty. I know from experience that indulging in live, vegan desserts can be yummy, nourishing, and healthy all at the same time. When our bodies are getting what they actually need and our brains are being fed, we cannot overeat the way we can on empty-calorie food. During this program, if you do splurge and eat a bunch of the healthy stuff, then so what! At the end of the day, you ate a head of cauliflower (disguised as popcorn), superfood chocolate shakes (that were also giving you vitamins), or some skin-nourishing, creamy avocados. Your body probably needed the vitamins they provided. You cannot say that while eating a bag of deep-fried chips, deep-dish pizza, or donuts.

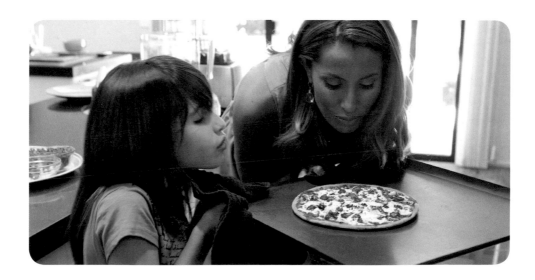

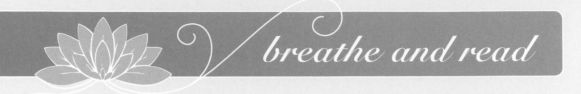

breathe and read

WHAT ABOUT PROTEIN?

I am frequently asked the question, "Where do you get your protein?" This is understandable because a common misconception about the vegan diet is that it is protein deficient. With knowledge and practice, you will find this is simply untrue. And because it is such a hotly debated topic, I feel that it's important to include a crash course in protein as you begin your cleanse.

The word "protein" means "to come first." Protein is made from amino acids and contains nitrogen as the distinguishing element, as well as carbon, hydrogen, and oxygen. Protein is needed for tissue growth and repair and for the formation of blood cells, antibodies, enzymes, hormones, and neurotransmitters. It is a source of food energy and helps in the water-electrolyte balance of the body.

Though Americans get plenty of protein, disease is rampant. Amino acids (there are twenty-two aminos, eight of which must be obtained from food or supplements) start being destroyed at 118 degrees Fahrenheit and are virtually all deactivated by 160 degrees. Cooking causes the proteins to coagulate and become denatured. This makes proteins less digestible and more inflammatory. Cooking food to slightly under 200 degrees causes leukocytosis, where leukocytes (white blood cells) that would be used to attack a foreign substance are called in to help digest food. The renowned Max Planck Institutes (comprising nearly eighty research organizations under that umbrella and doing groundbreaking work in life sciences research) have found that even small increases in protein consumption can decrease the body's ability to transport oxygen, which can be a factor in cancers. After we eat a cooked protein meal, white blood cells increase by as much as 600 percent. This signals that the immune system is trying to maintain homeostasis. The Max Planck researchers have discovered that a person only needs half as much protein as previously believed when protein is consumed in its raw state. When eating raw or living foods, the need for protein decreases from about 70 grams daily to approximately 35 grams daily. When life is very stressful, the need for protein increases.

Protein digestion uses up about 70 percent of its caloric content. Proteins are broken down into amino acids through an enzyme catalyzing process called proteolysis, usually with the help of hydrochloric acid. Excess protein can overload the lymphatic system's ability to cleanse itself. An excessively high-protein diet can contribute to heart disease, high blood pressure, arthritis, gout, osteoporosis, and various disorders of the kidneys, liver, and prostate.

The media's encouragement to eat more dairy, eggs, and meat is fueled by those industries that want you to buy their products. Although these foods are high in protein, they are also high in fats and represent the captivity, suffering, and exploitation of animals. Certainly humankind survived off animals during many times of hardship and necessity, but that practice is no longer needed for most people. As we will explore further, eating lower on the food chain exposes us to less herbicide and pesticide residue. Also, consider the strength and power of oxen, racehorses, and gorillas—all of whom eat a vegetarian diet.

The bottom line: there is some protein in all foods. Protein is present in the nucleus of almost every cell of every life form on earth in the form of DNA.

Complete vegetable proteins include almonds, bee pollen, blue-green algae, buckwheat, chlorella, garbanzo beans (chickpeas), hemp seeds, pumpkin seeds, quinoa (pronounced *keen-wah,* quinoa is the only grain that is a complete protein), sesame seeds, soy foods (tempeh, tofu, edamame), spirulina, and sunflower seeds. All nuts (including almonds, listed above) except filberts are complete proteins, containing an average of 10 to 15 percent protein.

Other good protein sources are alfalfa, amaranth, apricots, avocados, bananas, beans, berries (goji berries and Inca berries are great sources), broccoli, brussels sprouts, cabbage, carrots, cherries, cauliflower, coconut, corn, cucumbers, dates, durian, eggplant, sprouted grains, grapes, green beans, green leafy vegetables (including arugula, chard, clover, collards, dandelion greens, kale, lettuce, mustard greens, parsley, spinach, turnip greens, watercress), lentils, maca, melons, millet, mung beans, okra, sun-cured olives, oranges, papayas, peas, peaches, pears, peppers, protein powders (made from hemp seeds, pea protein, brown rice protein, or spirulina), sprouts, seaweeds, summer squash, sweet potatoes, tomatoes, and zucchini.

Vegetables have a higher percentage of protein per calorie than fruit (about four times as much of their total calorie content). On average, fruit has about as much protein as mother's milk. Most fruits contain protein in amounts from 4 to 10 percent of their total calorie content. Here are a few examples of the amount of protein based on the total calorie content:

- Almonds 12 percent
- Broccoli 45 percent
- Buckwheat 15 percent
- Cabbage 22 percent
- Honeydew 16 percent
- Kale 45 percent
- Pumpkin 15 percent
- Spinach 49 percent
- Walnuts 13 percent
- Watercress 84 percent
- Zucchini 28 percent
- Seaweed 5 to 30 percent, depending on type

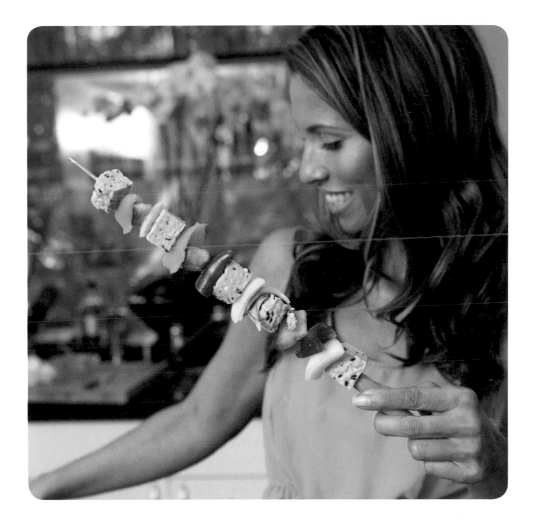

Once you begin to incorporate the principles and recipes I have shared throughout this book, the many benefits will be your firsthand experience. The rejuvenation begins the moment you begin indulging only in foods that come from a plant, bush, or tree and release anything that has been overly tampered with and is potentially blocking your flow. Make it an adventure! Visit your local farmers market or nearby community garden for fresh produce. Explore the vegan whole foods at your local health food store or coop to discover the many vegan options available. For an immediate selection of vegan restaurants in your area, visit www.happycow.net.

Three weeks of eating healing, whole, living foods will nourish and transform you on every level—body, mind, and soul—by recalibrating and rejuvenating every single cell in your body. You are already perfect. Now is the time to make food choices that support the full expression of that perfection.

CHANNELS OF ENERGY AND LIGHT
week one

Opening to Receiving

Echoing chapter 1, the subtle channels of energy and light that run through our bodies, connecting us with the source of life, are known as the *nadis* in the healing traditions of the ancient yogis. This week, allow yourself to be carried on the current of *ida*, the feminine and receiving principle that is one of the three primary forces of the *nadis*. *Ida* corresponds to the left side of the body and the right side of the brain. It is the introverted, lunar *nadi* that is associated with the sacred river Ganga in the yogic consciousness.

CUSTOMIZING YOUR SUPERSTAR PLAN
week one

For many, the idea of trying a vegan diet is a brand new consideration, and for others, a vegan lifestyle is already a way of life. No matter where you find yourself on the spectrum, this part of the program can be fine-tuned to address and enhance your own personal needs. Most importantly, I strongly encourage you to stay away from chemicals and processed foods. When you use whole foods—especially fresh veggies, whole grains, seeds, and fruits—as the mainstay of your meals, your health and beauty will improve more quickly.

FOR THE BEGINNER

If eating vegan is new to you, this is your week to explore and enjoy new foods, textures, and tastes while benefiting your health in numerous ways. Believe it or not, there is almost always a vegan substitute for anything that you might be missing or craving, such as the vegan pancakes and "grilled cheese" sandwich you will soon have an opportunity to try.

FOR THE INTERMEDIATE

If you are vegetarian, here is your chance to explore a 100 percent nondairy vegan diet for the next three weeks. And if you are already a vegan, how can you take it to the next level possible? Have you tried going gluten free to free up more energy and heal any lingering digestive or inflammatory issues? The next step for you could be to release all refined flours and refined sweeteners. Have you become addicted to agave nectar or the vegan dessert section of your grocery store? Have you lost touch with more grounding foods such as root vegetables like rutabaga and turnips? Are you including enough fruits and vegetables in your diet without relying on too many processed vegan "junk foods"? Remember: we are aiming for as close to an unprocessed, whole food diet as we can get. Your goal is always to increase the quantity of organic produce and whole foods in your current regimen, shift to gluten-free foods, and relinquish all refined sugars. If you are already on a healthy, gluten-free, sugar-free vegan diet, then your next step is to begin to incorporate more raw foods into your diet.

FOR THE ADVANCED

Eating a diet that consists entirely of living foods that are brimming with vitamins, minerals, enzymes, and other life-giving constituents is one of the greatest secrets of superstars everywhere, whether that superstar is on the big screen or a shining light living in the next apartment. If you are already a 100 percent live food vegan, you know the extraordinary difference this commitment has made to your health and life. Now, I have an interesting invitation for you: consider taking the opportunity to go back to a vegan lifestyle for one week. What I have found is that doing this cultivates a compassionate flexibility and gives way to valuable personal insights, all without forfeiting the commitment to a plant-based diet.

If you choose not to stray from your live food regimen for one week, then look to see how you can further refine your present lifestyle. Are you overly rigid about your eating habits? If so, how can you soften? Are there any addictions or sabotaging patterns that you can take steps to release during the cleanse, whether an addiction to a chemical substance, an emotional state, a relationship pattern, or some other way that you might be currently out of alignment with your true self? When you talk about a live food diet with others, do you find yourself helping and inspiring others or judging and making recommendations with a little too much urgency? If you can relate to that, just know that it's never too late to become a flexitarian—at least in heart and mind.

FOR EVERYONE

From beginner to advanced, there are action steps and inner reflection activities throughout the twenty-one days to support you in reaching for the next-highest level of diet and lifestyle choices.

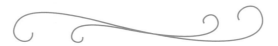

PREPARING FOR YOUR SUPERSTAR GLOW
week one

Are you ready now for your most luminous self? The following simple steps will provide you with the core information, inspiration, and suggestions for self-care that will give you a solid foundation for making the most of your twenty-one-day process.

STEP 1

It's movie time! Visit www.meatrix.com and watch all three parts of *The Meatrix,* an informative animated film totaling approximately ten minutes. For an even more sobering and effective run at this, try watching *Meet Your Meat,* a short documentary narrated by Alec Baldwin that is pretty convincing, especially if this is not your first time around the vegan block.

STEP 2

In Rainbeau's Reading Room, read the following sections to further support your journey:

1. Go Organic on page 344.
1. Understanding pH Balance on page 348.
2. The Essential Nutrients on page 355.

STEP 3

Each morning, begin your day by reviewing the applicable daily Toolkit section. There you will find suggestions for body, mind, and spirit—from daily recipes to action steps—that will put you in alignment with your highest potential and more. Commit to incorporating at least one suggestion that speaks to you. You are creating a new, strong foundation made of commitment, compassion, and self-love. To help you achieve total inner and outer balance, the daily Toolkit options will quicken the healing and nourishment of your cells and the release of cravings and self-destructive patterns.

STEP 4

Daily exercise increases oxygen in the body, stimulates blood circulation, energizes and moves the lymphatic system, and encourages detoxification. For best results, schedule your *ra'yoKa* and *Yoga for Beauty* poses and any other exercise for the same time each day to help your body acclimate to these potentially new habits.

STEP 5

Be attentive to your energy level and need for rest, especially during the first two weeks of the cleanse process. If you find yourself feeling tired, go ahead and take a nap (or at least a short break), while simultaneously trusting that your body is at work utilizing all of the nutrients and resources you have blessed it with.

STEP 6

Remember, this is your time to *relax*, *release*, and *rejuvenate*. The more peace and well-being you experience, the more you will see that this is a program you can return to over and over again. You can use it as needed to peel away layers of time, stress, and unhealthy choices, and reveal more and more of your personal radiance.

To remove the past, we align with the now.

That's all there really is anyhow.

To become who we are, we move toward the core.

Love is really what we came here for.

Everything we need is already within.

RECOMMENDED SHOPPING LIST
stocking your superstar glow pantry

Most of the ingredients in this recommended shopping list are readily available today, even in many of the conventional grocery store chains. However, you can also purchase certain items online and sometimes at a discount. *Note: With select items, I have included my favorite brands in parentheses. Just do the best you can and choose things YOU like, as everything I am sharing is merely a suggestion.*

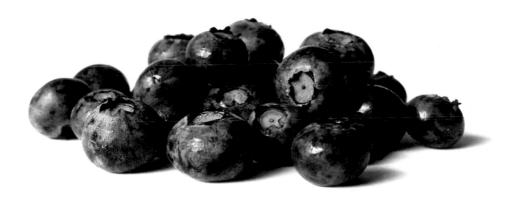

FRUITS & VEGGIES

- Avocados
- Bananas
- Berries, such as blueberries, strawberries, blackberries, raspberries
- Cauliflower
- Celery
- Coconuts (especially young Thai coconuts, the "white" coconuts due to the green husks being shaved off)
- Cucumbers
- Eggplant
- Greens: dark leafy greens, such as arugula, chard, collard greens, kale, spinach
- Jicama (crispy, sweet root vegetable; looks like a large potato and is easy to eat raw)
- Mushrooms, portobello or shitake
- Parsnips
- Peppers (red, yellow, green)

- Romaine lettuce
- Sun chokes
- Seasonal fruit, such as apples, apricots, oranges, papayas, peaches, plums, watermelon
- Tomatoes, cherry
- Yellow squash
- Zucchini

Note: As much as possible, base your choices on what is in season and organic. And if certain types of fruits and vegetables spark your interest, talk to your produce person at your favorite store. They might give you a sample to try or special order hard-to-find foods.

GRAINS

- Black rice (remember: the darker the grain, the higher the mineral content)
- Brown rice
- Buckwheat noodles (100 percent buckwheat)
- Corn tortillas
- Daiya brand dairy-free cheeses or other dairy alternatives (make sure they do not have casein, which is a milk protein)
- Millet
- Oat groats *(note: oats, oat groats, and oat flour are not gluten free; omit if gluten sensitive)*

- Quinoa (technically a seed, quinoa is used as a grain—light and nutty tasting)
- Rice noodles
- Sprouted grain or gluten-free bread or bagels
- Wild rice

NUTS

Your choice of raw …
- Almonds
- Brazil nuts
- Cashews
- Macadamias
- Pecans
- Walnuts

SEEDS

- Chia seeds (from the chia plant, these tiny seeds are an ancient superfood, rich in omega-3 fatty acids and extraordinarily high in antioxidants)
- Flax seeds
- Pumpkin seeds
- Sesame seeds
- Sunflower seeds

Note: Nuts and seeds are sensitive, so it may be ideal to store them in the refrigerator until soaking, sprouting, or using.

BEANS & LEGUMES

- Black beans
- Chickpeas (garbanzo beans)
- Lentils
- Tempeh (fermented soybean cake), as well as other soy alternatives to meat (and even pasta)

HERBS & SPICES

- Basil
- Cayenne
- Celtic sea salt
- Chili powder
- Cilantro
- Cinnamon
- Cumin
- Curry mix
- Dill
- Garlic
- Ginger
- Italian mix that includes a variety of herbs (look for unsalted and add Celtic sea salt instead)
- Mint
- Nettles
- Parsley
- Peppercorns (white or black)
- Rosemary

SWEETENERS

- Agave (nectar or syrup of the agave cactus plant)
- Coconut sugar
- Dates
- Raw honey
- Maple syrup
- Raisins
- Stevia (a sweetener extracted from the leaves of the stevia plant; 200 times sweeter than sugar and does not raise blood sugar)

CONDIMENTS

- Apple cider vinegar, unpasteurized
- Bragg Liquid Aminos (liquid protein concentrate derived from non-GMO soybeans; not fermented or heated and gluten free, it is a healthy replacement for tamari and soy sauce)
- Coconut oil, organic extra virgin (recommended brand: Divine Organics)
- Miso, unpasteurized
- Mustard
- Nama shoyu (raw, unpasteurized soy sauce) or wheat-free tamari
- Nutritional yeast
- Olive oil, organic extra virgin, stored in a dark glass bottle and away from heat
- Salsa
- Tomato sauce or pizza sauce

SUPERFOODS & SPECIALTY ITEMS

- Acai (pronounced *ah-sigh-ee*, acai is the berry of a special Amazon palm tree that is remarkably high in antioxidants)
- Aloe vera juice/pulp
- Almond butter, raw
- Bee pollen
- Blue-green algae
- Cacao powder (Cacao is the bean that chocolate is made from. In its raw state, it contains more antioxidant flavonoids than red wine, green tea, or blueberries.)
- Cacao nibs (from the cacao bean)
- Camu camu (a tropical fruit that is similar to a cherry and grows deep in the Amazon rain forests; is known to be extremely high in a potent form of vitamin C and phytochemicals)
- Chlorophyll
- Goji berries
- Golden berries (also called Inca berries, these tart and nutrient-dense berries are high in carotene and bioflavonoids)
- Green tea, yerba maté, and/or chai, organic
- MSM powder (methylsulfonyl-methane is a naturally occurring form of dietary sulfur found in fresh raw foods and rainwater)
- Maca (powder derived from the root of an herbaceous plant native to the high Andes of Bolivia and Peru; recommend brand: HealthForce Nutritionals*)
- Moringa powder (a green powder from the moringa tree with a nutty aroma; high in vitamin C and potassium)
- Noni (the fruit of a flowering shrub native to the Pacific islands; a magical fruit very high in vitamins, minerals, and antioxidants)
- Protein powder (recommended brands: Sunwarrior or HealthForce Nutritionals)
- Royal jelly
- Seaweed, such as dulse (a reddish-brown seaweed, slightly spicy and great in soups and on salads), kelp
- Spirulina (recommend brand: HealthForce Nutritionals)

Dr. Jameth Sheridan of HealthForce Nutritionals launched the standard known as TruGanic: the purest, hard-core quality standard for sourcing and production, significantly beyond "organic." Products must pass rigorous tests to verify they are 100% pesticide, insecticide, herbicide, irradiation, and GMO free (ZERO detectable).

- Sun-cured olives
- Sun-dried tomatoes
- Superfood trailmix (recommended brand: Divine Organics Bliss Mix)

- UliMana Truffle Butter (a premade truffle butter made from cacao butter, cacao powder, agave, vanilla beans, and Celtic sea salt)

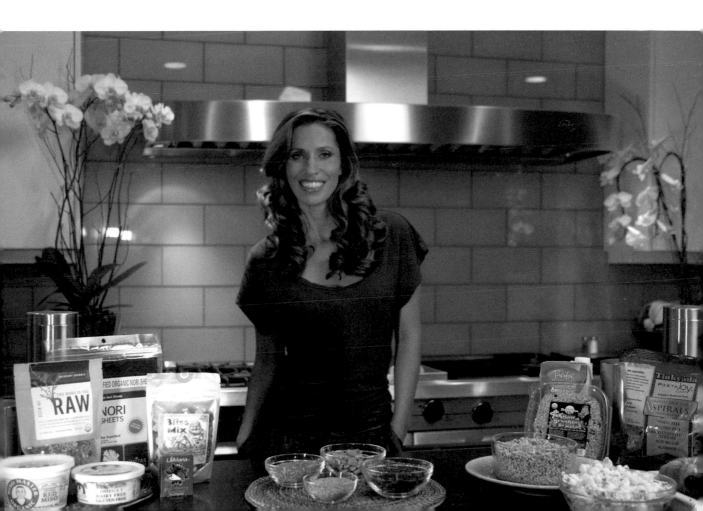

"If someone wishes for good health, one must first ask oneself if he is ready to do away with the reasons for his illness. Only then is it possible to help him."

—HIPPOCRATES

FOODS TO ELIMINATE
to achieve your superstar glow

REFINED WHITE SUGAR
Sugar is highly processed and weakens the immune system. Because of its acidity, it also leaches calcium from the body and can contribute to candida (yeast overgrowth) in the body. Choose instead: raw honey, dates, agave nectar, and real maple syrup (grade B preferred). These sweeteners are mineral rich and minimally processed.

REFINED FLOURS (ESPECIALLY BLEACHED WHITE FLOUR)
Flour contains gluten, an allergen for many people, with strong addictive qualities. Refined flours are also generally devoid of nutrients and not nourishing for the body. Foods containing gluten can slow down your digestive system, create bowel issues, and decrease energy levels. Choose instead: brown rice, 100 percent buckwheat, quinoa, gluten-free spelt, and sprouted grains (which are whole foods). *Note: Regular spelt does contain gluten.*

DEEP-FRIED FOODS
During the three-week cleansing period, fried foods are completely unnecessary. Overcooking food, as is the case with frying anything, greatly diminishes the nutrient content in the food. Once ingested, fried foods also create free radicals that are damaging to the body and encourage premature aging.

When we remove chemicals and saturated fats from the diet and reduce the production of free radicals, our body's natural ability to heal will accelerate. Fried foods include tempura, French fries, potato chips, and donuts. Choose instead baked or dehydrated foods.

ALL ANIMAL PRODUCTS

Think of food as a conduit of energy. Animal foods contain the energy of the animals they came from. The yogic tradition believes that ingesting animals that have been mistreated in any way brings that energy inside you. When we are cleansing out toxins, taking in this type of dense energy is counterproductive to revealing your radiance. Additionally, the manner in which animal products are processed employs harmful, toxic agents such as GMOs (genetically modified organisms), antibiotics, hormones, and sadly, parasites and types of bacteria that must be cooked to kill. Animals and their by-products usually come from unhealthy and diseased sources. Animal products include chicken, fish, steak, pork, lamb, shrimp, mussels, ice cream, yogurt, milk, cheese, sour cream, and butter. Alternatives include meat substitutes created from mushrooms, soy, coconut, nuts, seeds, and eggplant; fats like coconut oil, raw olive oil, nut butter, seed cheeses, and vegan butter; and coconut-based or nut-based milks, yogurts, and ice creams. Watch out for hidden or inconspicuous ingredients containing animal products or by-products such as casein, milk powder, lard, and of course milk and cheese.

FAST FOODS

When eating out, choose restaurants that offer raw, whole foods or simply find restaurants with salad bars. Many restaurants now have vegan options available. Search the Internet to try something new and support the vegan-friendly restaurants in your area.

REGULAR TABLE SALT

Table salt is chlorinated and processed in a manner that strips away the life-giving minerals that naturally occur in salt. Choose instead: Himalayan or Celtic salts, sea kelp, dulse, or nama shoyu (raw, unpasteurized soy sauce).

OVERLY PROCESSED, REFINED, PACKAGED FOODS

Instead of foods laden with preservatives, choose organic, whole, fresh, local foods and produce.

CAFFEINE

If you are a coffee drinker, there are truly delicious alternatives! Try yerba maté (especially satisfying when made with a French press and adding nondairy milk or creamer), raw chocolate shakes, or even ground dandelion root as a tea to help you wean off coffee/caffeine. If you drink black tea, I suggest that you switch to green tea (it has been said that "green tea gives the spirit a place to rest"), chai made with rooibos, or another lightly caffeinated or decaf tea. I like chai because the black tea is combined with digestive and thermogenic (fat-burning) herbs such as cinnamon and clove—just make sure it's dairy-free.

ALL CHEMICALS PRESENT IN YOUR LIFESTYLE

For the first week, if you drink alcohol, imbibe only organic, sulfite-free wine, top-shelf tequila, or organic gluten-free options for drinks (beer contains gluten, for example). If you smoke marijuana for medical purposes, make sure it's truly organic and use only a vaporizer. If you smoke cigarettes, limit to no more than one per day and only if it is an organic cigarette made from chemical-free tobacco. Smoking is a part of some sacred traditions, but it was originally about the prayer. Unfortunately, without ritual and due to the great overabuse of sacred plants, these substances are now contaminated; smoke is toxic and creates organ stagnation, which gets in the way of cleansing. So, if you must use these crutches, do so with the intention of finding replacements that are healthier. Step by step, feed yourself with life-giving choices rather than those that are fogging and numbing to the mind, body, and emotions. There are some herbs that are truly clearing, and alcohol was once referred to as "spirits"—that's because in small amounts and taken intentionally, it can lift the spirit. At least ask yourself, "Can I let go of this for right now?" You can do anything for twenty-one days, right?

Three More Helpful Tips

Yogis say it's best to eat your largest meal when the sun is highest in the sky. That's when the digestive enzymes are at full peak, and so is your energy. The internal fires are stoked and are ready to burn the energy (food and nutrients) you supply them with.

Although I am not super-rigid about following the exact times, we can't do anything well on an overly full stomach, like make love, sleep, or practice yoga. Learn how to give your body a break as you make some of these activities a higher priority.

If you do eat late, make sure you spend more time before eating in the morning. It's said that a nightly fast of twelve to fifteen hours is great for the system. Eat when you're hungry, but be mindful of "eating to live" rather than "living to eat."

Fluids can dilute the digestive fires, especially cold fluids, ice, and other cold foods. In yoga, because we like to build heat to detoxify the body, I recommend practicing on an empty stomach and not eating for thirty minutes before or twenty minutes after a session. Consider using this same guidance concerning fluids while eating; make it a practice as much as possible. I personally break this rule while drinking warming digestive aids, and if you must have water while eating, choose lemon water without ice.

The Invitation

Rather than focusing on what you might be giving up by eliminating these habits for the next three weeks, open your arms wide to embrace all you are clearing the way to receive—increased vitality, inspiration, creativity, joy, and well-being.

THE LIVER KICK ...
and other liver tonics

The liver is an integral part of your health and wellness, the great detoxifier of the body. It has many essential functions, making the proteins needed to produce blood and hormones, creating enzymes and other chemicals we need to facilitate the communication of cells, and of course facilitating digestion. It also metabolizes fats, sugars, and dead cells. Without our liver, we would not live.

Liver flushes, like this Liver Kick, are used to stimulate elimination of waste from the body, increase bile flow, and improve overall liver function. They also help purify the circulatory and lymphatic systems.

The liver is known as one of the most important organs of the body, second to the heart. In addition, it's considered the parent of the heart in Asian medicine, so that means to open and connect in our hearts, we must release the stagnant toxic energy in our livers, which governs anger and depression.

When releasing liver bile, toxins, and stuck emotions, it's important that we use our powers of visualization and intention to move the energy through and out of us gracefully, rather than giving in to frustration. Remember that "stuff" must come up in order to move out.

SPECIAL NOTE REGARDING MORNING LIVER FLUSHES

At the beginning of each day (reflected on each day's Schedule page), I recommend that you do the *liver flush of your choice*. This means that you can choose the beverage you most enjoy and/or alternate between them. Here are the three simple flushes I recommend:

1. The Liver Kick (most potent choice) described next.
2. The ACV Tonic on page 330, slightly easier on the taste buds than the Liver Kick.
3. A simple (yet powerful!) cup of hot water and lemon.

LIVER KICK

INGREDIENTS

- Juice of 3 or 4 lemons
- Juice of one orange (optional)
- 1 tablespoon of extra virgin olive oil or coconut oil (high quality, organic)
- 1 inch of ginger
- 1 clove of garlic (I do this on the days I know it will be okay; also the cleaner we are, the less we retain foul smells.)
- *Optional ingredient:* HealthForce Nutritionals Liver Rescue (supports liver detoxification and regeneration; especially effective during a cleanse, yet gentle enough to take on a daily basis)
- *Recipe variation:* To the basic Liver Kick recipe add equal parts of lemon grass, fennel, and fenugreek seed.

DIRECTIONS

Drink the liver flush drink first thing in the morning at least one hour before breakfast and fifteen to twenty minutes before drinking anything at all, even water.

NOTES

You may "flush" the liver up to thirty days, cycling off for three days for every ten on. You can continue to eat and drink regular amounts live foods in this cleanse while you do so.

If you have experience cleansing or you have already completed a full cycle of The 21-Day SuperStar Cleanse, *you may want to enhance Week Three with a gall bladder flush for one to seven days—that is, during days fifteen to twenty-one.*

I strongly recommend doing this as much you can. Make lemons your best friends and have them stocked, but make sure to brush your teeth after consuming them because lemons are strong. Following the guidelines provided here will greatly enhance the overall results of this program.

DAY ONE **SCHEDULE**

QUICK REMINDER: The Toolkit section is the all-important anchor for this twenty-one day cleanse. What you will find here are the daily virtues, featured recipes, aligning action steps, yoga and *ra'yoKa* poses, and mantras that will enlighten your body, uplift your consciousness, and turn you into a superstar!

7:00 AM	DAWN GLOW TONIC	
	Liver Kick (page 94)	

8:00 AM	BREAKFAST	
	Jumpstart Chia Breakfast (page 325)	

10:00 AM   YOGA POSE OF THE DAY
ra'yoKa Sequence of the Day
Option: Take a walk or go to the gym

12:00 NOON   LUNCH
Recipe of the Day: Grilled Chees-ini Sandwich (page 308) with a side salad
Kombucha tea

1:00 PM   SELF-TLC
Option: Create a vision board (collage) of your goals
Option: Contemplate today's action step for Aligning with Your Ultimate Purpose

4:00 PM	DINNER
	Queen (Quinoa) and King (Kale) Salad (page 319)

6:00 PM	GET YOUR GLOW ON
	Put your legs up the wall and listen to music or read for fifteen minutes

AS DESIRED	SNACKS & DESSERTS
	3 dates with almond butter (or whole almonds inside each date) and a dash of cinnamon

7:00 PM	DUSK GLOW TONIC
	Relaxing herbal tea. My favorites are nettles, mint, and ginger.

SUPPLEMENTAL RECOMMENDATION

Take one to three enzymes (as suggested according to brand). Always include with each cooked meal to aid digestion and cellular cleansing.

DAY ONE **TOOLKIT**

Virtue of the Day: Humility

With humility, we can allow ourselves to see the limitations of some of our ways of thinking, doing, and being. True humility invites an openhearted honesty with oneself that is a powerful starting place for making important changes. In this sense, humility is a doorway to freedom, allowing us to make new choices. Let humility guide you today in seeing a limitation so that you can be free to make a new choice, especially one that relates to food.

Action Step of the Day: Aligning with Your Ultimate Purpose

Shift habits today. Deviate from your normal routine by exploring some fresh, stimulating activity you have, always wanted to try, or that a friend told you about. For example, you could ...

- Pick up the book you have wanted to finish (or start)
- Write a poem, a blog post, a short story
- Compose a song
- Take a new yoga class or dance class
- Go for a walk and take in the surroundings and beauty of your area
- Join some friends or local naturalists on a hike through a park

Take this day to *set yourself free* by exploring different activities the world has to offer you.

RECIPE OF THE DAY: **GRILLED CHEES-INI SANDWICH**

Enjoy this vegan variation on the classic grilled cheese sandwich.

INGREDIENTS

- ⅓ cup water
- 4 teaspoons nutritional yeast
- 1 tablespoon oat flour; can be a spoon of oats whizzed in the blender (*note: oats and oat flour are not gluten free; omit if gluten sensitive*)
- 1 tablespoon fresh lemon juice
- 1 tablespoon tahini
- 2 teaspoons tomato paste or ketchup
- 1 teaspoon cornstarch
- ½ teaspoon onion granules
- ⅛ teaspoon garlic granules
- ⅛ teaspoon turmeric
- ⅛ teaspoon dry mustard
- ⅛ teaspoon Celtic sea salt
- 4 slices gluten-free bread

DIRECTIONS

1. Place all the ingredients minus the bread in a saucepan and whisk together until the mixture is smooth. Bring to a boil.
2. While stirring constantly, reduce the heat to low. Cook until the cheese sauce is thick and smooth, then remove from heat.
3. Cover one side of each piece of bread with the cheese sauce.
4. Grill the sandwiches in a skillet or toaster oven and serve with some veggies on the side.

For a quick grilled cheese, try just grilling the bread on a griddle or skillet with coconut oil, sprinkle with your preferred type of Daiya cheese, and place one piece of the bread on top of the thoroughly melted Daiya. Add whatever else you might like in the sandwich or as a side.

DAY ONE **TOOLKIT**

ra'yoKa Sequence of the Day: *Seated Vertical Wave*

Today is about introspection—cultivating inner awareness and connecting with yourself. Begin in *Virasana* (shown below) or *Sukhasana* (easy cross-legged position) with your arms to the side of your body. Inhale and lift your chest up, with the arms following the chest, reaching back and up. Extend through long wrists and out through the fingers. On your exhale, round the back and shoulders to release the neck and spine. Think about collecting energy from the earth and drawing it into the body and up into the next inhale. Repeat this cycle three to six more times.

Mantra of the Day: I AM LOVE, I AM WORTHY,

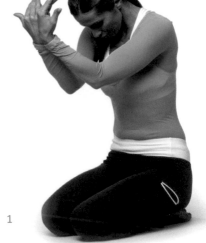

1

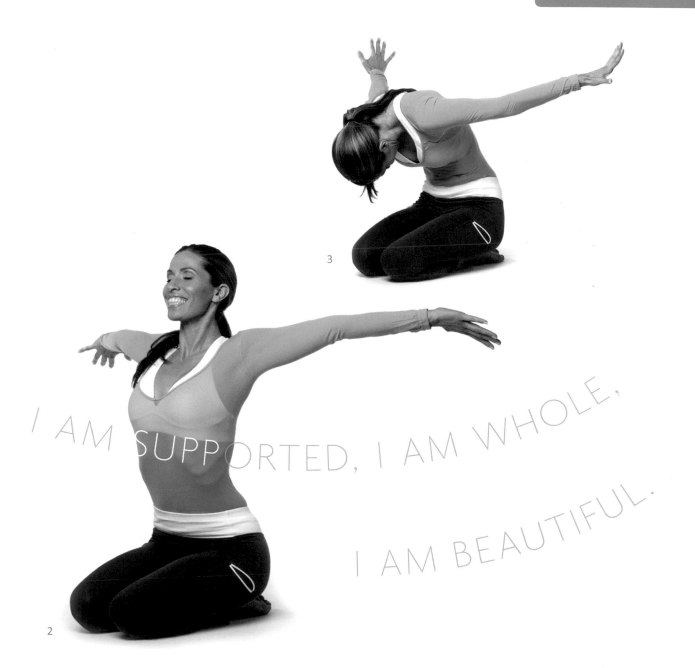

3

2

I AM SUPPORTED, I AM WHOLE, I AM BEAUTIFUL.

DAY TWO **SCHEDULE**

7:00 AM   DAWN GLOW TONIC
Hot Apple Cider Tea (page 334) or liver tonic of your choice

8:00 AM   BREAKFAST
Toasted sprouted grain bread with coconut oil and raw honey spread

10:00 AM   YOGA POSE OF THE DAY
Option: *Yoga for Beauty* Pose of the Day
Option: Try a dance class to embrace your adventurous side

12:00 NOON   LUNCH
Recipe of the Day: Vegan Pizza (page 313)
Lemonade (page 334)

1:00 PM   SELF-TLC
Option: Read an inspiring book passage
Option: Contemplate today's action step for Aligning with Your Ultimate Purpose

DAY **2** ★

4:00 PM | DINNER

Black Bean Vegan Burger Patties with a side of salad (page 306)

6.00 PM | GET YOUR GLOW ON

Treat yourself to a luxurious Beauty Bath; see the Superstar Skin section on page 274 to find your head-to-toe glow.

AS DESIRED | SNACKS & DESSERTS

1 flax cracker with almond butter and raw honey
1 to 2 handfuls raw nuts

7:00 PM | DUSK GLOW TONIC

Hot Apple Cider Tea (page 334)
Option: fresh squeezed lemon in water with a dash of cayenne and maple syrup

---

SUPPLEMENTAL RECOMMENDATION

Support your cleanse with HealthForce Nutritionals Liver Rescue.

DAY TWO **TOOLKIT**

Virtue of the Day: *Generosity*

Often when we think of generosity, we think of a willingness to give. As important a trait as that giving quality is, generosity is actually so much more! It also implies a fullness of being and a readiness to share the overflow, whether that is an overflow of money, energy, creativity, or love. On this second day of your twenty-one-day journey, let yourself be inspired by daydreaming about how you will share the new abundance of energy and inner resources that you are calling forth within yourself.

Action Step of the Day: *Aligning with Your Ultimate Purpose*

Rather than turning on the TV tonight, spending time online, or distracting yourself in some other way, take time to write about your goals, commitments, and feelings. Do you know who you really are? Who would you like to be? What can you do for the next three weeks to realize your highest self?

RECIPE OF THE DAY: **VEGAN PIZZA**

Because I want you to realize that there are always healthier versions of everything, we're going to kick off the cleanse with a crowd pleaser.

INGREDIENTS—TOPPING CHOICES:

- 2 large tomatoes, cut in half and sliced
- 2 garlic cloves, crushed
- Handful of fresh basil leaves
- Daiya cheese, mozzarella (optional)
- Grain sausage substitute (optional)
- 1 container pizza sauce or regular tomato sauce (or even salsa)

For extra "veggie love" try chopped onions, eggplants, zucchini, and peppers.

INGREDIENTS—CRUST:

2 wheat-free crusts can be found in most grocery stores; you'll usually want enough for other people and leftovers. Rice crust is great, and cornmeal is yummy too, yet usually contains some wheat.

DIRECTIONS

1. Preheat the oven to 425° F.
2. Take the crusts out of wrappers.
3. Spoon on evenly the pizza or tomato sauce or salsa
4. Place the tomatoes and sprinkle on garlic and basil and cover with Daiya cheese.
5. Use the veggies and experiment with a grain sausage on one or, if you love them, both of the crusts.
6. Place in middle of oven for about 10 minutes—and standby while shredding romaine lettuce to serve on the side.
7. For the extra veggies, grill the chopped onions in coconut oil until clear and then add the rest of the cubed veggies.
8. Let sit and cool until needed before topping pizza.
9. Play it cool as friends beg to join the cleanse.

DAY TWO **TOOLKIT**

Yoga for Beauty Pose of the Day: Child's Pose

Starting in a "table" position (on your hands and knees), move your hips back onto your heels. Rest your hips there with the tops of your feet flat on the floor. Arms come back toward your hips and rest on the floor, with your head resting on the mat. Rest, breathe, and soften your hips, jaw, head, back, and ears. Let your head and arms release fully and breathe. Take at least five nourishing breaths.

Mantra of the Day: Let Go and Let Flow

However you perceive the divine, in whatever shape, form, or essence, allow yourself to have the support of this infinitely loving force. If you have any uncomfortable feelings brewing, such as anger, frustration, doubt, or fear, know that you don't have to hold on to them or handle them on your own. Offer any painful feelings or negative beliefs up to source … and let in the idea that everything will work out for your highest good … always.

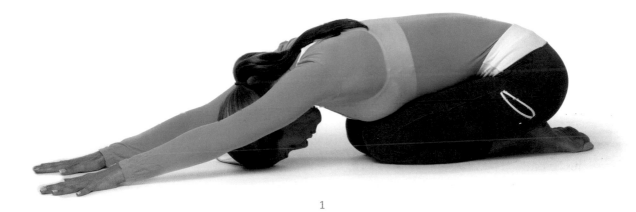

1

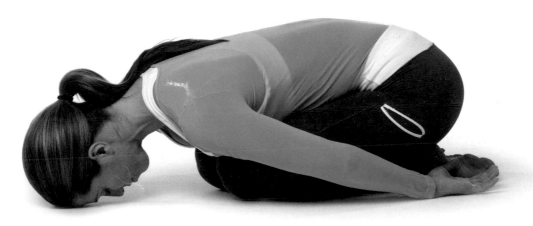

2

DAY THREE **SCHEDULE**

7:00 AM DAWN GLOW TONIC
Start with liver tonic of your choice
Then try nettles tea or fresh mint tea with some yerba maté
and feel tons of energy

8:00 AM BREAKFAST
Superfruit Smoothie (page 336)

10:00 AM YOGA POSE OF THE DAY
Option: *ra'yoKa* Sequence of the Day
Option: Take a brisk walk with a friend

12:00 NOON LUNCH
Enjoy Creamy Avocado Kale Salad (page 318)

1:00 PM SELF-TLC
Option: Give yourself an eco-pedicure (with nontoxic nail polish).
See the 28 Beauty Rituals section on page 370 for helpful tips.
Option: Contemplate today's action step for Aligning with
Your Ultimate Purpose

DAY 3 ★

4:00 PM — DINNER

Recipe of the Day: Vegetable Tempeh Kebobs Skewer
(page 313)

6:00 PM — GET YOUR GLOW ON

Give yourself a facial. Make a nourishing mask of whole
plain yogurt and lavender essential oil. If you don't have
yogurt, try papaya!

AS DESIRED — SNACKS & DESSERTS

1 to 3 flax crackers with raw almond butter or coconut butter
and raw honey or organic, vegan jelly.

7:00 PM — DUSK GLOW TONIC

Try a digestive tea that gets things moving, such as ginger,
mint, or chamomile

SUPPLEMENTAL RECOMMENDATION

Try taking a few capsules of acidophilus to culture the system. I like to take one
of these at night. My favorite brand right now is Boulardii MAX by Advanced
Naturals, which also supports the immune system. However, you can find
many others, such as dairy-free Bio-K+ (a fermented soy probiotic).

DAY THREE **TOOLKIT**

Virtue of the Day: *Kindness*

Treating ourselves with kindness is one of the most effective ways on earth to bring out our superstar glow—it is one of the most nourishing "substances" in existence. Treat yourself with the utmost kindness today, especially in the privacy of your own thoughts about yourself and the words you say out loud about yourself.

Action Step of the Day: *Aligning with Your Ultimate Purpose*

With all the news of different toxins found in packaging materials, like BPAs (the chemical compound bisphenol A) in plastics and the toxic dyes in paper, glass jars are making a comeback as the preferred storage containers. Plastics leach chemicals, and aluminum can oxidize juices or add a metallic flavor to foods, but glass jars are the perfect vessel for safely storing foods. If you don't have any glass jars, find a mason jar that you can designate as your special container. Keep and reuse a few food jars—pickles, almond butter, jam … all of these jars are ready to find their new purpose! An added bonus is the ability to see the quality of the containers of the food you buy (a pickle jar, for example) as an investment in toxin-free kitchenware. Green your life and kitchen by reducing packaging, reusing packaging, and of course, recycling.

RECIPE OF THE DAY: **VEGETABLE TEMPEH KEBOBS SKEWER**

This dish is a perfect merging of distinctive flavors and satisfying textures. Enjoy!

INGREDIENTS

- 1 package tempeh
- 8 wooden skewers (soak in water to make skewering easier)
- 4 cubed portobello or shiitake mushrooms
- ½ zucchini (cut in half lengthwise)
- ½ red onion cut into ½-inch chunks
- ½ red pepper, large dice
- ½ yellow pepper, large dice
- 8 cherry tomatoes

INGREDIENTS—MARINADE:

- 6 tablespoons wheat-free tamari
- 1 cup apple juice
- ¾ cup orange juice (2 oranges)
- 4 to 8 cloves garlic, minced
- 2 tablespoons Dijon mustard
- 3 tablespoons minced fresh rosemary, or 1 tablespoon dried
- 1 cup liquid coconut oil or olive oil (½ cup for marinade, remaining for vegetables)

DIRECTIONS

1. Cut the tempeh in half.
2. Place the tempeh into a pot with the marinade and simmer for 30 minutes.
3. Cube simmered tempeh into 4 cubes (for a total of 8) after it cools.
4. Add oil to marinade and marinate vegetables for an hour or more.
5. Create kebobs using vegetables and 1 cube of tempeh per skewer.
6. Grill 5 minutes on each side and serve warm or at room temperature.

DAY THREE **TOOLKIT**

ra'yoKa Sequence of the Day: *Horizontal Wave*

Begin on all fours. Exhale back onto the balls of your feet into an active Child's Pose. Your toes are tucked under, hips are sitting on the heels, back is rounded inward, arms are stretched forward, and your fingertips are connecting to the ground. Empty yourself as you sit back toward your feet (allowing them to spread and positively affecting the whole body) and draw your belly into the spine. Inhale, roll forward and feel every vertebra of the spine get massaged and stimulated. Let the movement clear the spine and body. Exhale as you return to the starting position. Repeat these movements three to six more times.

Notice how today's pose is the physical equivalent of the mantra of the day provided below—with the pose taking you down, in, back up, and then out and forward.

Mantra of the Day:

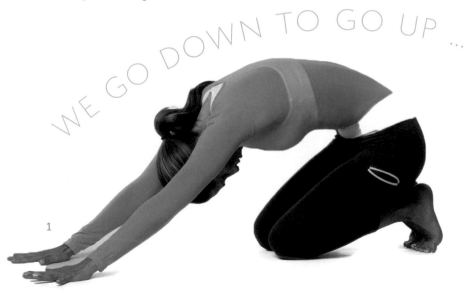

WE GO DOWN TO GO UP ...

1

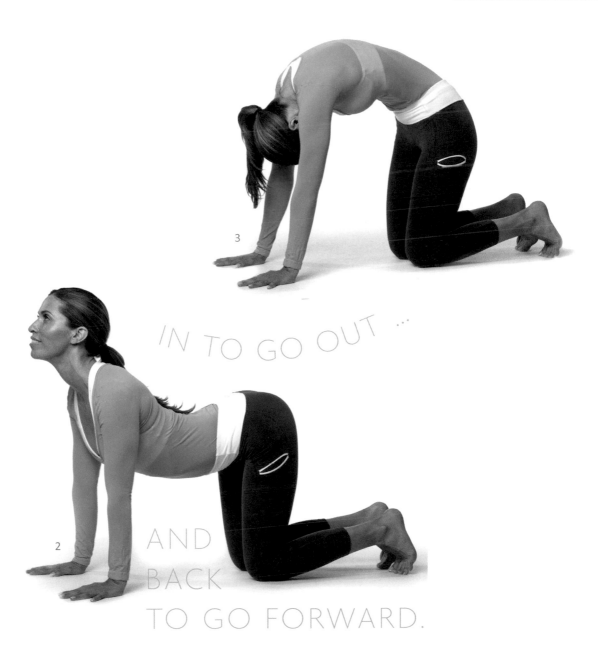

3

IN TO GO OUT ...

2

AND
BACK
TO GO FORWARD.

DAY FOUR SCHEDULE

7:00 AM   DAWN GLOW TONIC
Start with liver tonic of your choice
Yerba Maté Latte (page 337) or decaffeinated tea of choice

8:00 AM   BREAKFAST
Recipe of the Day: Banana-Topped Vegan Pancakes (page 324)

10:00 AM   YOGA POSE OF THE DAY
Option: *ra'yoKa* Sequence of the Day
Option: Try a local Tai Chi or martial arts class

12:00 NOON   LUNCH
Kelp Noodle Stir-Fry (page 309)
Iced yerba maté tea or hot lemonade

1:00 PM   SELF-TLC
Option: Practice conscious breathing (pranayama)
Option: Contemplate today's action step for Aligning with
Your Ultimate Purpose

DAY 4 ★

4:00 PM	DINNER
	Easy Vegan Quesadillas (page 307)

6:00 PM	GET YOUR GLOW ON
	Play! Turn on upbeat music and just dance!

AS DESIRED	SNACKS & DESSERTS
	Flax crackers with creamy garlic dip—a blend of macadamia nuts, garlic, lemon, some rosemary, and water as needed

7:00 PM	DUSK GLOW TONIC
	Fresh coconut water or Divine Organics coconut water in a glass bottle

SUPPLEMENTAL RECOMMENDATION

Are you having cravings for certain foods or beverages? Write them down in your journal, and notice if the process of moving them from your body to the page creates any kind of shift in your cravings.

DAY FOUR **TOOLKIT**

Virtue of the Day: *Zeal*

Today we are dusting off a word that may not be used very often, but one that holds the power to launch our greatest dreams—*zeal*. Zeal has heat to it! It is a merging of passion and enthusiastic action toward a specific outcome. If you're feeling a little tired on this fourth day of your cleanse, spend a few minutes thinking about something that stirs feelings of warmth, enthusiasm, and excitement for you. There you will find your zeal!

Action Step of the Day: *Aligning with Your Ultimate Purpose*

Find a new route to your main destination today. As you are going through many changes and transformations—including an exploration of new ideas on food, lifestyle, and mind-set—take the spirit of change just a little further today and map an entirely different path to work, school, or other primary destination. Every time we try something new, we create new neurons in our brain that make us smarter.

If you can, choose one other day during this three-week process where you take an entirely different *mode* of transportation to work or other end point. Try taking public transportation, carpool with a coworker or friend, ride your bike, or maybe even see if you can skip the roads altogether and work virtually for one day. Our choices of today are tomorrow's past, so let's concentrate on building a cleaner, healthier future for everyone.

DAY **4**

RECIPE OF THE DAY: **BANANA-TOPPED VEGAN PANCAKES**

This recipe is proof that health, beauty, and indulgence blissfully coexist. Feel free to try a gluten free ready-made flour mix and nondairy substitutes.

INGREDIENTS

- 1¼ cups almond or rice milk
- 1 tablespoon lemon juice
- 1 tablespoon vegetable oil
- 1 tablespoon maple syrup, plus extra for serving (grade B has more minerals)
- ½ cup buckwheat flour
- 1 teaspoon baking soda
- ½ cup flour or flour mix, choice
- ½ teaspoon salt
- 2 bananas, thinly sliced

DIRECTIONS

1. Mix all the wet ingredients together in a small bowl.
2. Mix all the dry ingredients together in a slightly bigger bowl.
3. Add the wet to the dry and stir just enough to mix.
4. Heat a large nonstick skillet over medium-high heat.
5. Spoon the batter onto the skillet and cook for about a minute and a half or until the bottom side is golden brown and the top has small bubbles.
6. Repeat until you run out of batter, then serve with banana slices and maple syrup.

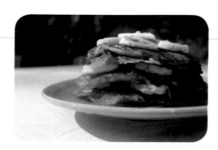

DAY FOUR **TOOLKIT**

Mantra of the Day:

I CONNECT IN POWER, HARMONY, AND BALANCE AT MY CORE.

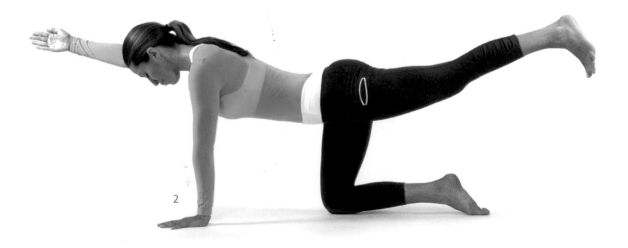

DAY 4

Healing In Stretching
~~ra'yoKa Sequence of the Day:~~ _Core Pulses on Knees_
dance

Begin on your hands and knees, making sure that your wrists are directly under your shoulders, even with the mat and each other, and shoulder width apart. Your knees should be directly under your hips, hip width apart. Inhale, lift the left leg back; fully extend the left leg and make sure it is straight, strong, and parallel to the ground. On your next inhale, lift the opposite arm (the right arm) up and hold it out in front of you. Extend all the way through your fingertips. Take a deep breath. On the next exhale, draw in through your core. Bend your left knee in toward your abdomen, while you also bring your right elbow in toward your knee to hug all the way in. Inhale and extend the arm forward and the leg back to its original position. Repeat this six times. Always use one breath, one movement. Switch sides; extend the right leg back and bring the left arm forward this time, repeating the sequence.

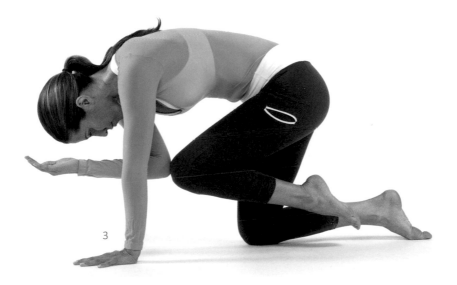

3

DAY FIVE **SCHEDULE**

7:00 AM   DAWN GLOW TONIC

ACV Tonic (page 330) or liver tonic of your choice

8:00 AM   BREAKFAST

Morning Miso Soup (page 316)

Option: Superboost Shake, if soup seems funny (page 336)

10:00 AM   YOGA POSE OF THE DAY

Option: *Yoga for Beauty* Pose of the Day

Option: Kick up the pace—go for a run, walk, or jog

12:00 NOON   LUNCH

Recipe of the Day: Coconut Curry with Bok Choy (page 307),
served on a bed of brown rice with a side salad

1:00 PM   SELF-TLC

Option: Try a therapeutic spinal massage or other desired
type of massage—perhaps a massage chair (they are
everywhere now)

Option: Contemplate today's action step for Aligning with
Your Ultimate Purpose

DAY **5** ★

| 4:00 PM | DINNER |
| | Soba Pasta with Tahini Miso Sauce (page 311) and a side of steamed broccoli and raw tomato slices with Celtic sea salt and raw olive oil |

| 6:00 PM | GET YOUR GLOW ON |
| | Try a *ra'yoKa* DVD or download and explore an integrative yoga fusion |

| AS DESIRED | SNACKS & DESSERTS |
| | Piece of fruit and handful of raw almonds |

| 7:00 PM | DUSK GLOW TONIC |
| | Ginger-mint tea with whole peppercorns for a kick |

SUPPLEMENTAL RECOMMENDATION

Try eating a piece or two of raw vegan chocolate.

DAY FIVE **TOOLKIT**

Virtue of the Day: *Purity*

Purity is an exquisite experience of mind and body in which we are freed up from physical, emotional, or mental states that can seriously bog us down (for example, illness, shame, or guilt). Today, sense the purity you are allowing to come forth within yourself, especially from the food choices you're making this week. Feel the innocence and light within each cell of your body.

Action Step of the Day: *Aligning with Your Ultimate Purpose*

Researchers and medical doctors alike have published studies confirming that the lining of our stomachs regenerates every five days. Well, congratulations are in order because for these first five days of your cleanse, you have been giving your body only the most healing and nutritious foods as the optimal building blocks of the ever-blossoming and regenerating "new you." This is only the beginning of the momentum we are cultivating together on this journey of freeing the body's natural healing processes and abilities.

Of course, the stomach is one part of a powerhouse area of the body. Expanding your perspective outward, think of the solar plexus, navel (or belly button), and stomach—all intimately connected to other major organs of detoxification: the liver, gallbladder, and pancreas. This is the home of the third chakra, sometimes called the radiant gem. What will support the optimal functioning of your core right now? Even as you thoroughly enjoy your cooked vegan recipes and breads, be sure to eat high-fiber foods, especially water-rich fruits and vegetables. Also, acidophilus products are excellent for digestion problems and to obtain and maintain a healthy amount of good bacteria (beneficial intestinal flora). A gentle massage helps too. In fact, you can try a gentle self-massage right now. Place your left hand on your right side and go up,

DAY **5**

RECIPE OF THE DAY: **COCONUT CURRY WITH BOK CHOY**

The blending of coconut and curry could be considered ambrosia of the gods … and goddesses.

INGREDIENTS

- ½ medium onion
- 1 bunch bok choy
- 1 clove garlic
- 8 ounces tempeh
- ¾ cup coconut milk
- 2 tablespoons coconut oil
- 1 cup diced heirloom tomatoes
- ½ teaspoon curry powder
- 1 teaspoon garam masala
- 1 teaspoon grated ginger (optional)
- Pinch of Celtic sea salt to taste

DIRECTIONS

1. Sauté tempeh in coconut oil in skillet until browned on all sides.
2. Dice the onion and the crunchy stalks of the bok choy and add to the skillet to cook until soft.
3. Chop and set aside the bok choy leaves.
4. Blend the garlic clove, curry, garam masala, ginger, and tomatoes in a blender or food processor until smooth.
5. Once onions and bok choy are soft, add tomato mixture and chopped bok choy leaves to the skillet.
6. When leaves are wilted, add coconut milk; cook until heated through.
7. Season to taste with salt and serve over brown rice or quinoa— and of course your favorite side salad for the enzymes.

DAY FIVE TOOLKIT

across your abdomen, and then down, moving in the same direction as your large intestine (in a clockwise path) and connecting to what's there. This will assist with digestion and metabolism. In the Asian healing traditions, the element of Fire resides in the solar plexus and functions as the furnace of vital energies, giving expression to the radiant sun of our personality, will power, and creativity. For healing, regeneration, and balance, connect with the Fire element by enjoying short sunbathing sessions, lighting candles at home, or visualizing the color yellow in all its vibrancy.

Yoga Pose of the Day: *Downward-Facing Dog Pose*

Find equanimity today as you begin on your hands and knees on the floor, with your knees below your hips and your hands placed slightly ahead of the shoulders. Root down through your palms with fingers facing forward, and curl your toes underneath. On an exhale, lift your hips toward the ceiling as you straighten your legs, at first keeping the knees and arms slightly bent and the heels lifted as you push through the balls of your feet. Drop your head as you lengthen through the spine, elongating your neck to create space between your shoulders. Begin extending through strong legs to straighten, but take care not to lock the knees, and more importantly, keep the back straight. With firm arms, press your palms into the floor and roll the arms out as you lift along your inner arms from the wrists to the tops of your hips. Breathe deeply and hold for one to three minutes as your body surrenders to this all-over body stretch and strengthener. When finished, bend your knees to return to the floor on an exhale and come to rest in Child's Pose.

Mantra of the Day:

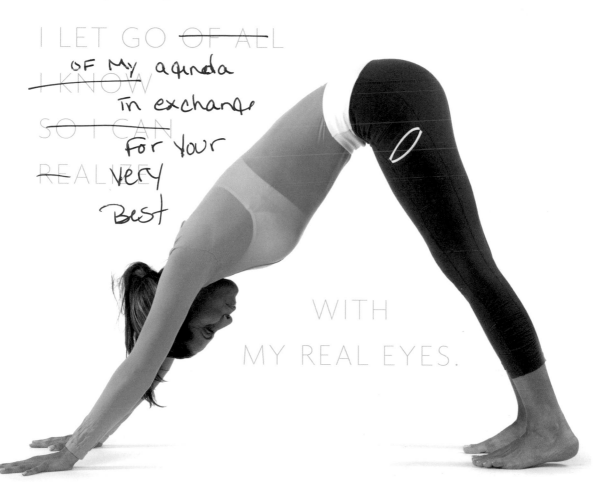

I LET GO ~~OF ALL~~
OF My agenda
~~I KNOW~~
In exchange
~~SO I CAN~~
for Your
~~REALIZE~~ very
Best

WITH
MY REAL EYES.

DAY SIX **SCHEDULE**

7:00 AM DAWN GLOW TONIC

Start with liver tonic of your choice

Then enjoy a nice dairy-free (and possibly caffeine-free) chai

8:00 AM BREAKFAST

Comforting Whole Groat Oatmeal (page 325)

10:00 AM YOGA POSE OF THE DAY

Option: *ra'yoKa* Sequence of the Day

12:00 NOON LUNCH

BBQ Tempeh & Greens Sauté (page 305)

Pomegranate juice or organic red wine

1:00 PM SELF-TLC

Option: Listen to a guided visualization

Option: Contemplate today's action step for Aligning with

Your Ultimate Purpose

4:00 PM	DINNER	
	Recipe of the Day: Red Grape Vegan Tacos (page 311)	
6:00 PM	GET YOUR GLOW ON	
	Try a local Tai Chi or martial arts class	
AS DESIRED	SNACKS & DESSERTS	
	Waste not—enjoy leftovers from the week	
7:00 PM	DUSK GLOW TONIC	
	Green Clean Juice (page 333)	

SUPPLEMENTAL RECOMMENDATION

Hydration is your friend—a key to flowing energy and supple skin! Remember to drink eight glasses of water a day. The water source should be good and better than just treated tap water from a big chemical factory. Look for spring water sources, and it's great if it can be bottled in glass. Try flavoring with cucumber, lemon, mint, and even a touch of Celtic sea salt. You could also add a splash of raw honey or stevia to enjoy it even more.

DAY SIX TOOLKIT

Virtue of the Day: Dignity

When we treat ourselves with dignity, we are acting as the superstar we truly are. From this place of self-respect, we are uplifted and inspired to make choices that are in alignment with our innate potential. If a physical or emotional craving arises today, tap into the power you can access when you own your worthiness—and with dignity, choose not to give in to the craving.

Action Step of the Day: Aligning with Your Ultimate Purpose

Since many of us spend much of our time indoors, having high-quality indoor air is a must for optimal health and restoration. Health is wealth, and I do recommend having a good air filter that can circulate the air with antibacterial essential oils like lavender or eucalyptus. However, having clean air doesn't have to require buying an air filtering system—nature is happy to lend a hand. NASA did a study to find out which plants were best to filter the air of the space station, and here is their top list:

- English ivy (*Hedera helix*)
- Peace lily (*Spathiphyllum* "Mauna Loa")
- Chinese evergreen (*Aglaonema modestum*)
- Bamboo palm or reed palm (*Chamaedorea sefritzii*)
- Heartleaf philodendron (*Philodendron oxycardium*, syn. *Philodendron cordatum*)
- Elephant ear philodendron (*Philodendron domesticum*)
- Rubber plant (*Ficus elastica*)

Welcome a few of these green lovelies into your home and *breathe free*!

DAY 6

RECIPE OF THE DAY: **RED GRAPE VEGAN TACOS**

Recipe contributed by one of our favorite Superstar Cleanse participants, Aisha

INGREDIENTS—MAIN SALAD FOR THE TACOS:

- ½ large jicama, peeled and thinly sliced (about 1½ cups)
- 1 cup cilantro leaves and stems, finely chopped
- ½ cup red seedless grapes (organic), halved
- ½ avocado, diced
- 1 lime, juiced
- 1 tablespoon olive oil (optional)
- 1 finely diced jalapeño
- Dash of smoked paprika
- Salt and pepper to taste

INGREDIENTS—TORTILLAS AND CONDIMENTS:

- 4 corn or rice tortillas
- 1 cup fresh chopped tomato salsa (chopped tomato, onion, garlic, and cilantro)
- 1 can black beans, drained and warmed on stovetop for a few minutes
- 1 cup guacamole (chopped avocado, tomato, lime juice, cilantro, salt and pepper to taste)
- Vegan sour cream
- Vegan shredded cheese, such as Daiya cheese

DIRECTIONS

1. Combine all main salad ingredients in a large bowl and toss well.
2. Chill for at least a half hour to allow flavors to marinate and mix.
3. Warm tortillas on the stove or in the oven, sprinkling with vegan shredded cheese (cheese optional).
4. Assemble the tacos to your liking and enjoy with friends!

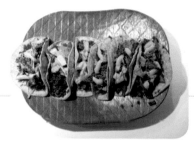

DAY SIX **TOOLKIT**

ra'yoKa Sequence of the Day: Flowing Forward Wave

Begin in Downward-Facing Dog. Remember, just as with all yoga poses, if you are not breathing, you've gone too far. Begin with your breath ... always. Come to the tops of the feet—the tops of the toes. Moving forward on your exhale, uncoil the spine vertebra by vertebra. Round your back and look in toward your belly button. Continue drawing in as much as you can, as you round the spine. Come forward into a plank position with a rounded spine. Lower slowly down toward the floor. Once you have lowered toward the ground, push yourself back up to a Cobra Pose. Keep your toes tucked. Gently push down through your front palms and lift your hips off the ground, if you feel inclined to do so. Pull your chest forward, hands back toward the feet (near the hips). A slight bend in the elbow and wrists directly underneath your shoulders will lengthen your body forward out of your lower back and open the chest. Reverse out of Cobra by uncoiling the back bend one vertebra at a time, staring with the neck (home of the highest vertebrae), and moving again into Downward-Facing Dog.

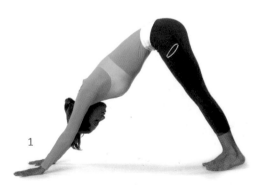
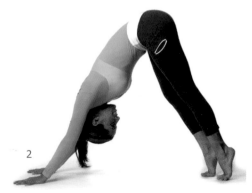

1

2

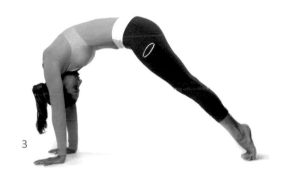

3

Mantra of the Day:

WHEREVER WE GO, THERE WE ARE.

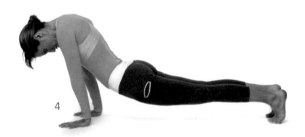

4

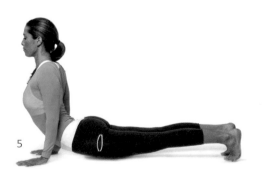

5

DAY SEVEN SCHEDULE

7:00 AM	DAWN GLOW TONIC
	Hot Apple Cider Tea (page 334)
8:00 AM	BREAKFAST
	Delightful Fruit Salad (page 318) with avocado added
	Sprinkle with your favorite superfood powders (for example, cacao, maca, or lucuma)
10:00 AM	YOGA POSE OF THE DAY
	Option: Yoga Pose of the Day
	Option: *ra'yoKa* Sequence of the Day
12:00 NOON	LUNCH
	Recipe of the Day: Black Bean Vegan Burger Patties (page 306) with a side of fresh herb salad
	Fresh coconut water or Divine Organics coconut water in glass bottle
1:00 PM	SELF-TLC
	Option: Journal about what you have experienced so far ... physically, emotionally, and mentally
	Option: Contemplate today's action step for Aligning with Your Ultimate Purpose

4:00 PM	DINNER
	Wild Rice Harmony (page 320) with a side of Easy Kale Salad (page 319)

6:00 PM	GET YOUR GLOW ON
	Try *Yoga for Beauty: Dusk* DVD or download to help wind down for the night

AS DESIRED	SNACKS & DESSERTS
	Moringa Bliss Balls (page 328)
	Option: Indulge guilt free with UliMana Truffle Butter with a sprinkling of cacao nibs

7:00 PM	DUSK GLOW TONIC
	Peppermint tea with raw honey and lemon

SUPPLEMENTAL RECOMMENDATION

Today's supplement is holy basil. This plant creates a euphoric and almost intoxicating feeling as it opens the mind and heart. I have used the plant fresh and in teas, but a great way to try it is in enteric-coated capsules. Break open about five capsules in your mouth and perhaps drink something nice to follow the bitter taste. Enjoy feeling open, alive, and probably a bit more psychic.

DAY SEVEN **TOOLKIT**

Virtue of the Day: Love

On the seventh day of your twenty-one-day program, you are invited to rest in the arms of love. For every triumph and stumble you may have experienced during this first week, love is the response from yourself that you deserve most of all. Take a deep breath in and sense the love coursing through your entire body and being ... the love that is lighting up the world around you.

Action Step of the Day: Aligning with Your Ultimate Purpose

If Week One of your SuperStar Cleanse meal plan is going well overall, but you're having trouble letting go of certain foods, beverages, or other habits, it may be wise to give your home a fresh start too. Our homes are an extension of ourselves and can often be an insightful reflection of our internal environment. For instance, toxins stored in the body might be mirrored to us in the external world, appearing as the clutter we see in our bedroom or closets. We are most influenced by the things, events, and people that are closest to us; therefore, it's important to bring some attention and awareness to how we can refresh our immediate surroundings, cultivating greater inner and outer harmony. The ancient Chinese healing art form known as Feng Shui is a brilliant system for inviting harmony, balancing the flow of *chi* (vital life force energy), and regulating energetic influences.

To best support your superstar glow, consider applying some of the principles of Feng Shui to your bedroom, a space that is meant to be a temple of nourishment, rejuvenation, and romance. Most days, our own bedroom is the last setting we see before we fall asleep and the first setting we see upon waking. Do you like what your eyes are drinking in at these important moments? There are easy remedies for transforming your private sanctuary. First, take out all the items that create clutter or negativity, whether that clutter is visual,

RECIPE OF THE DAY: **BLACK BEAN VEGAN BURGER PATTIES**

This vegan version of the ever-popular burger is earthy, grounding, and delectable!

INGREDIENTS (MAKES 6 BURGERS)

- 2 cups black beans (soaked overnight for eight hours, rinsed, and drained)
- 2 carrots, grated
- ½ cup dry rolled oats (*note: oats are not gluten free*)
- 1 tablespoon olive oil
- ½ teaspoon each of your preferred spices: cinnamon, cumin, coriander, chili powder, onion powder, black pepper or cayenne pepper (¼ teaspoon of the peppers)
- 1 teaspoon Celtic sea salt

DIRECTIONS

1. Preheat oven to 300° F.
2. Grate the carrots, then add oats, ¾ cup of the beans, your spices, and the olive oil—mixing all together in the food processor.
3. Spoon mixture into a mixing bowl and then fold in the rest of the whole reserved beans. Wet your hands and then form into 6 medium-sized patties.
4. Bake at 300° F for 40 minutes, turning once halfway through.
5. If preferred, prebake for 30 minutes and cook for final heat on the grill until lightly browned.
6. Add to sprouted wheat buns and enjoy. Perfect for vegan cookouts in the spring. Serve with a side or fresh herb salad, which makes an excellent addition to anything you're eating (there is a salad I eat so often that I've given it my own name—Rainbeau's Favorite Herb Salad on page 320).

DAY SEVEN **TOOLKIT**

spatial, or energetic (think EMFs). It may seem radical, but consider removing items such as an unused TV, exercise equipment, office- or work-related items, and storage items, all of which can drain your energy and disrupt restful slumber. Even the neglected nooks and crannies in the rooms of our homes reflect those of the body, so don't forget to clean under the bed (which should be free of everything for restful and clear sleeping), the backs of closets, and those small drawers that are magnets for "stuff." Recall the saying "Take nothing but pictures, leave nothing but footprints," and find some of the freedom in simplicity. In this bustling consumer society, there can be a thin line between us owning our stuff and our stuff owning us.

So, as you are cleaning out your body, see how much more you can get out of *The 21-Day SuperStar Cleanse* by clearing out the bedroom and other living spaces. Let it be fun and easy. The options are plentiful; try getting rid of at least twelve things in each room of your house. As for the items that don't belong in the trash or recycling bins, you could organize a sidewalk sale or host a giveaway party where your friends receive the things you're ready to let go of, or donate items to your preferred organization. And once you have a new (or renewed) canvas to work with, enjoy decorating in ways that reflect the changes that are taking place within you—even if that is as simple as putting two single red roses on your bedside table(s), as everything in your boudoir should be in pairs.

One of the greatest benefits of cleaning and decluttering your living spaces is that it offers a tangible way to be honest with yourself in the discovery of your true needs and passions at this time in your life. And that is what the twenty-one-day program is offering you from the inside out as well. Do an Internet search to find and print out the *Bagua*, the Feng Shui map, and use it for further guidance in each room of your house—to strengthen the chi and flow of energy that will support your inner environment.

ra'yoKa Sequence of the Day: *Hamstring Flow Sequence*

Begin in a low lunge, with your back leg flat on the floor extended behind you (start with whichever leg you wish). Your front knee is in line with the ankle (do not over-extend your knee past the ankle). Your front thigh is parallel to the floor. Glide forward; lengthen the chest as you bring it forward. Bring your shoulders down and back. Lengthen up and out during your inhale. Exhale; draw your body in toward the core. Uncoil forward while you straighten your front leg. Take deep, long breaths, pausing gently at the end of each exhale and inhale, allowing one breath for each movement. Repeat on each side at least six times.

Mantra of the Day:

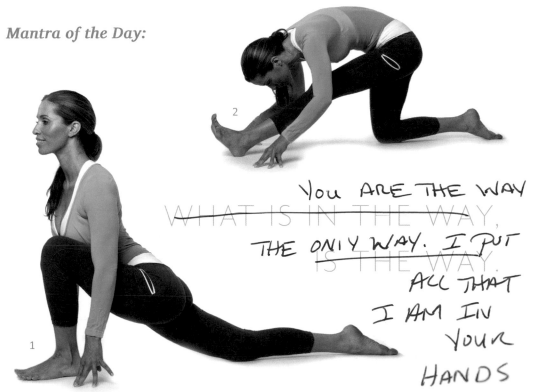

~~WHAT IS IN THE WAY IS THE WAY.~~

YOU ARE THE WAY, THE ONLY WAY. I PUT ALL THAT I AM IN YOUR HANDS

137

ILLUMINATIONS
week one

Finding Your Dreams in the midst of this cleanse

What I have discovered for myself is that it takes practice,

self-realization, and determination

To awaken day after day with a purpose and a passion that

aligns us with our destiny

It takes knowing that regardless of how many negative reasons there

are for doubting,

If we believe that the sky is limitless and that we can

do it, we can dream it.

I find my dreams when I let go,

Close my eyes,

Listen to nothing but the sound of my breath

And feel.

From that place, I can feel what experiences or things excite me,

What makes my heart beat faster,

And inspires me.

I do my best to live on the edge of what is as real and as

tangible as possible,

While always reaching for the stars,

One dream and step at a time.

♥ You lead me to the desires with in my heart when I feel release Control & Surrender to you

I choose Joy In every circumstance Because my existence goes way beyond My life here on earth.

I am eternal because of your GRACE

REFLECTIONS
discovering yourself anew

Writing in your journal or on your computer gives your the supreme gifts of self-inquiry and self-expression. You are now immersed in a simple yet profound process: one of making food choices that are more and more in alignment with the person you are becoming—the person you know you were born to be. I have found that engaging in regular segments of reflective writing is one of the greatest tools for integrating who we are today with the one we are becoming, both of which deserve our loving attention. To help you get into the flow of writing, the questions below are offered as touchstones for contemplation and meditation … and as writing prompts. Whether you write for five minutes or forty-five, I invite you to approach the page with kindness, curiosity, and honesty.

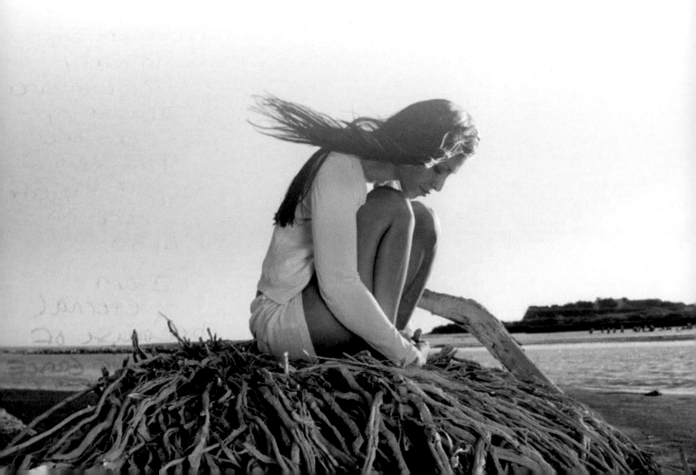

1. What was your experience of giving up animal products, fried foods, chemicals, or wheat? How did eliminating animal products from your diet make you feel, both physically and emotionally?

2. Did you experience any particular cravings this week? If so, were these cravings for specific foods or beverages, certain activities, or maybe a particular relationship? Did the cravings seem tied to an old emotional pattern? If so, were you able to identify and be with your underlying emotions? Also, did your cravings provide you with any new information or insights?

3. Were you met with limiting thoughts or beliefs this week? Such thoughts might have been: *I cannot go through with the program. I won't make it. I don't have any will power. I never complete anything.*

4. How easy or challenging was it to follow through with this week's recommendations and guidelines?

5. Did you incorporate any of the recipes, action steps, or inspirational tools such as the Daily Virtues and Mantra? If so, how did this self-care experience feel? If not, what prevented you from taking this time for yourself?

6. How did your body feel when you exercised this week?

7. Did you notice any changes in your sleep patterns?

8. What emotions did you experience? Did your moods change in noticeable ways?

9. Did you choose love over judgment this week? If your inner critic was active, there is always another chance to love yourself! You can start right now … it's only a matter of choosing. Choose one instance or area in your life where you can begin to practice unconditional love. Write down a specific step you can take within the next twenty-four hours to demonstrate that love.

WE ARE A
LANDSCAPE
OF ALL WE
HAVE SEEN.

—ISAMU NOGUCHI

CHAPTER 3

WEEK TWO: ACTIVATING WITH LIVE FOODS

The fast-acting power of live, uncooked foods—for healing, weight loss, and overall rejuvenation—often takes people by surprise. This was definitely the case with a friend who hired me to help him get in shape for an upcoming movie role. I had been teaching him yoga for some time, but now he had another goal to shoot for: to lose fifteen pounds in a short period of time. As we know, actors are accustomed to needing to morph their bodies to match the parts they play, sometimes gaining weight but more often needing to lose it. In the case of my client, much loved for his spirited, high-energy characters, he was interested in dropping the weight in the healthiest way possible. Not only did he want to look good—he wanted to *feel* amazing. When we started down this path, he told me he already ate healthy food and wasn't sure how he could really meet his goal without doing something extreme. When I outlined a cleanse overflowing with deliciousness, he was somewhat incredulous at first. With a meal planner that included foods like almonds, raw honey, avocado, raw chocolate, agave nectar, coconut sandwiches on buckwheat bread, decadent kale salads, superfood smoothies, and much more, it didn't look like any weight reduction plan he had seen before. "How can I eat so much and still lose weight?" he asked. A great question! The short answer was an easy one—the foods just have to be *living* foods. Technically, food is considered living or raw, with its enzymes in tact, when it has never been heated above 118° F.

When we eat whole, live foods that are nutrient-dense, enzyme-rich, and sparkling with life-enhancing electromagnetics, our bodies are able to digest those foods and absorb their nutrients with great efficiency. This is in contrast to the way our bodies respond to eating large amounts of cooked food, where the altered nature of the food, including the lack of enzymes, triggers an immune system reaction. In essence, the cooked food is seen as a foreign invader, which can get the dominos falling when the majority of our food is denatured in this way. Cellular inflammation, free-radical production, and congestion of the mucosal lining of the digestive tract are just a few of the common outcomes. It's important to reiterate here that I'm not suggesting that no cooked foods should be consumed; rather, it is a reminder of why it's so valuable to regularly give the body a break from cooked foods and aim for making more room for living foods in our kitchens and on our plates.

Giving his body a break from cooked food, this actor reached his fifteen-pound goal with complete ease in a matter of two weeks. In addition to delicious meals, he was doing Liver Kicks in the morning, scheduled a series of colonics, and dedicated three days to having blended foods only (which is where we are going in Week Three). Throughout the entire weight-loss cleanse, our focus was on keeping his metabolism running high and choosing foods and drinks that promote alkalinity—both essential for releasing weight. As important as his end-goal was to him, he actually enjoyed the process of getting to that point far more than he thought he would. And I believe that enjoyment is important to each of us, no matter what our goals or our timelines for getting there are. While we are in the process of enlivening our bodies (and eliminating that which makes us heavy, tired, toxic, sad, burned out, or sick), it makes sense that we would eat foods and engage in activities that are pleasurable, interesting, and awakening.

Sometimes we have relatively simple, targeted cleansing goals, like my client did for his movie. For the nonactors among us, there are weddings, family and school reunions, summer vacations, job promotions, and other events and occasions that are catalysts for wanting to look and feel like a million dollars. At other times, we may be prompted to make changes due to a health challenge or serious illness and the deep-down desire to reclaim total health. Whatever the case may be, I honestly cannot think of anything more important than the consistent rejuvenation and regeneration of our bodies by ridding ourselves of whatever is holding us back. When we lighten up in body, mind, and spirit, not only do we benefit, but our friends and beloveds also get to benefit from the warmth of our glow. Caring for ourselves gives us the energy, presence, and optimism to connect with them—and give to them—in truly inspiring ways.

SO LET'S GO DEEPER

This week is all about releasing the things that might be keeping you in a rut—feeling stuck, weighed-down, and maybe even fearful about what the future holds. The blockages in your life can be with your food choices, drugs (anything from Tylenol to cannabis), negative or toxic relationships, destructive patterns of behavior, and limiting thoughts about your abilities and your*self* in general. Our ego (or "small I") is content to keep bringing us back to the "comfort zone" of limitation because that is what it knows best. You may already know that these habits aren't serving you and wish to break them, and yet you might struggle against releasing them. This is a poignant struggle that almost every one of us can relate to in one way or another. Even when we start to make fantastic progress, there is a natural tendency for addictive cravings and the lure of old patterns to consume our attention (remember "the toxic relationship"?). But, no matter how long the patterns have held sway, it is never too late to free yourself from the past and move forward with your dreams.

As you start off on your Week Two adventure, know that no matter how much your ego wants to continue to define you (with its habits, rationalizations, and excuses), your deeper being wants to shine. And it *will* eventually win, because your birthright is perfect health and wellness. Like the snake shedding its skin, we are taking off old layers of egoic constructs so we can get to the core—the essence—of who we are. The day-by-day SuperStar structure of recommended meals and activities will support you to shed the dried-up layers of the past and discover the dazzling aliveness of yourself in the present. So keep reaching for and making the choices that are in alignment with your highest potential.

If we stay in our same old comfort zone, we'll simply stay the way we have been. In Paulo Coelho's book *The Alchemist*, there is a story demonstrating that successful people fall seven times but get up eight. This tells us that perhaps they are not failing but succeeding by taking an educated risk. This paints the picture that living just outside our comfort zone leads to change and success. Since all change comes from within, we must embrace the edge to experience transformation, healing, and the possible shift we are looking for. What we think, feel, eat, and do will all have direct effects on our inner alchemy. In other words, what we create inside impacts what we manifest on the outside. So together …

LET'S EMBRACE THE EDGE!

CHANNELS OF ENERGY AND LIGHT
week two

Upon the River of Giving

Focusing again on the *nadis*, the subtle channels of energy and light that run through your body, this is the week for consciously traveling along the current of *pingala*, the masculine and giving principle that is one of the three primary forces of the *nadis*. *Pingala* corresponds to the right side of the body and the left side of the brain. It is the extroverted, solar *nadi* that is associated with the river Yamuna, the largest tributary of the river Ganga.

Consciously call on the energy of *pingala* within you this week. Use your increased energy to give more, serve more, and make peace. This is the perfect time to get in touch with someone you haven't been in contact with for a while. Write a letter, make a phone call, send an email—be the one to reach out.

CUSTOMIZING YOUR SUPERSTAR PLAN
week two

Are you ready for more radiance? The opportunity of Week Two is to significantly increase the percentage of restorative living foods you eat each day. Assess where you are and what you feel prepared to do. What percentage of living foods will best serve you this week? Is it 100, 80, or perhaps 50 percent? You decide. My desire for you is that you set yourself up to win, feel great, have fun, and keep raising your awareness of what you are putting into your body and why.

This program is not about focusing on what is lacking or calorie counting. Go at *your own* pace and comfort level. As long as you continue to progress toward more vibrant, nutrient-dense food choices, you will achieve incredible results, as I have experienced myself and witnessed with hundreds of friends and clients over the years. With our easy-to-follow recipe and menu guide of live foods, you will know that beauty, health, and indulgence coexist.

FOR THE BEGINNER
If the vegan diet is already a huge step, take it to the next level this week. Completely cut out all refined flours this week. *Eat only whole foods* and keep it vegan.

FOR THE INTERMEDIATE
Let go of all starches, proteins, and refined foods. Good-bye rice, corn tortillas, beans, tempeh, and soy. Eat as many live foods as you possibly can. If the food you want is a vegan whole food (such as broccoli, cauliflower, or carrots), slightly cooked, steamed, or made into a soup, that is okay. Start getting excited, because the live foods will regenerate, clarify, and balance *everything*.

FOR THE ADVANCED

This is your time to go for it! Eat *only* living foods this week—nothing cooked. If you're already accustomed to eating a high-raw-foods diet, enjoy bringing even greater awareness to the food choices you make this week.

FOR EVERYONE

From beginner to advanced, the daily meal planners and the complete menu planner for Week Two will provide you with ideas, choices, and recipes that you can customize according to your tastes and your goals.

Helpful hint: Think of these recommendations as "cooking without fire." Instead, we are using our blenders, food processors, and dehydrators. We are using our marinades to nourish, lemons to oxidize, hands to massage and break down, and warm water to warm things up. Another way to view it is that we are cooking without killing.

PREPARING FOR YOUR SUPERSTAR CLEANSE
week two

Congratulations on completing one-third of this rejuvenation journey! I welcome you to potentially the most valuable part of the program. This week, you may be challenged to let go of your old ways of viewing yourself, life, and your old habits, especially with food. You are not alone in this evolutionary process. Let's do this together. Walk with me so that you can unfold without delay and fully inhabit your radiant potential. Let your true, beautiful self be your offering to the world.

STEP 1
Try a new live food recipe this week from your weekly menu, or from Rainbeau's Recipe Roundup.

STEP 2
Please read the following:
1. Ten More Reasons to Go Raw on page 356.
2. Five Flavors Theory of Traditional Chinese Medicine. See charts on page 366.
3. Eat the Rainbow chart on page 199.

STEP 3
Each morning, begin by reviewing the daily Toolkit section for the specific day of the cleanse. Commit to incorporating at least one suggestion, following your inner guidance and paying attention to the ideas and action steps that light you up inside.

STEP 4
As you journal about your live food experiences this week, think about how you can creatively incorporate more enzyme-rich foods into your daily lifestyle. What stores and farmers markets can you go to? When will you allot time for preparation? Who will be supportive of your process? Is there a live food event you could go to this week? Let yourself think, journal, and live outside the cooked food box.

STEP 5

What other live food resources can you look into as support? Are there any live food restaurants or potluck groups in your area? If not, consider starting one. If there are, go check them out and begin getting support and stocking up on living foods. Whatever you do, do not go hungry. If it's true that "we are what we eat," then when this journey is complete, do you want be radiant, fresh, light, beautiful, and alive, or cooked, refined, toasted, fried, smoked, and baked? Remember the goal.

Say it with me now ...

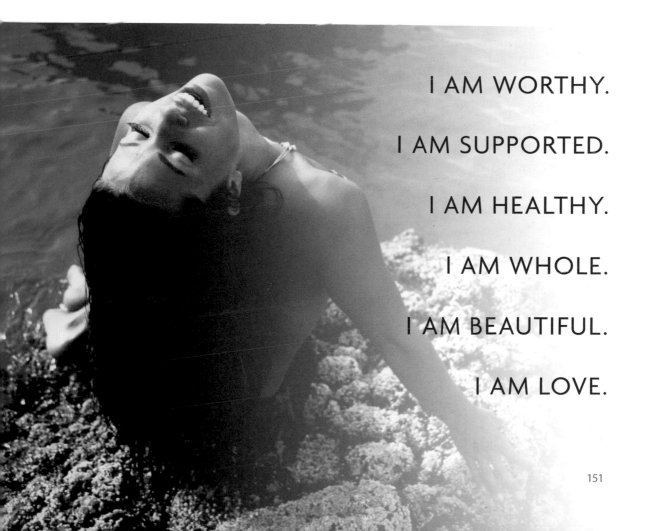

I AM WORTHY.

I AM SUPPORTED.

I AM HEALTHY.

I AM WHOLE.

I AM BEAUTIFUL.

I AM LOVE.

151

RECOMMENDED SHOPPING LIST
stocking your superstar pantry

As with the Week One pantry items, most of the ingredients in this recommended shopping list should be easy to find at your local grocery stores. If you already have these things, great! But stay abundant and ready to thrive and create. And remember to shop seasonally.

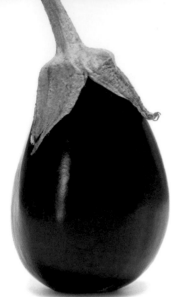

FRUITS & VEGGIES
- Avocados
- Bananas
- Berries, such as blueberries, raspberries, blackberries, strawberries
- Cauliflower
- Coconuts
- Cucumbers
- Eggplant
- Fruit, such as apples, bananas, lemons, limes, oranges, peaches, plums, watermelon
- Garlic
- Greens, including dark leafy greens, such as arugula, chard, collard greens, kale, spinach
- Jicama
- Kale chips (dehydrated and packaged)
- Onions
- Peppers
- Portobello mushrooms
- Romaine lettuce
- Tomatoes
- Yellow squash
- Zucchini

GRAINS, NUTS, & SEEDS
- Buckwheat
- Cacao nibs and/or beans
- Chia seeds
- Chickpeas (garbanzo beans)
- Flaxseeds
- Quinoa
- Nuts—your choice of raw almonds, Brazil nuts, cashews, macadamias, pecans, walnuts
- Sunflower seeds
- Wild rice

If you're short on time and can't make your own, have the following on hand:
- Raw crackers (such as flax crackers)
- Raw breads
- Raw cookies

HERBS & SPICES

- Basil
- Cacao powder
- Cayenne
- Celtic sea salt or Himalayan pink salt
- Cilantro
- Cinnamon
- Dill
- Garlic
- Ginger
- Licorice
- Mint
- Nettles
- Parsley
- Rosemary

SWEETENERS

- Agave
- Dates
- Raw honey
- Maple syrup
- Raisins

CONDIMENTS

- Apple cider vinegar, unpasteurized
- Bragg Liquid Aminos
- Coconut oil, organic extra virgin
- Miso, unpasteurized
- Mustard
- Nama shoyu or wheat-free tamari
- Nutritional yeast
- Olive oil, organic extra-virgin, stored in a dark glass bottle and away from heat
- Salsa

SUPERFOODS & SPECIALTY ITEMS

- Acai
- Aloe vera juice or pulp
- Almond butter, raw
- Bee pollen
- Blue-green algae
- Camu camu
- Chlorophyll
- Goji berries
- Green tea, yerba maté, and/or caffeine chai, organic (tea bags only)
- Lucuma (the powder of a sweet, tropical fruit from the lucuma tree; has a delicate caramel or maple-like flavor)
- Maca
- MSM powder
- Noni
- Protein powder, raw
- Royal jelly
- Seaweed, such as dulse, kelp, nori
- Spirulina
- Sun-cured olives
- Sun-dried tomatoes

DAY EIGHT **SCHEDULE**

7:00 AM	**DAWN GLOW TONIC**	
	Tea for good digestion, such as fresh mint, ginger, or cinnamon	

8:00 AM	**BREAKFAST**
	1 smoothie, shake, or fruit salad (add avocado if desired)

10:00 AM	**YOGA POSE OF THE DAY**
	Option: *Yoga for Beauty* Pose of the Day
	Option: Take a trip to the gym or go for a long, brisk walk

12:00 NOON	**LUNCH**
	Have an amazing salad with everything raw—such as mixed greens, chopped and marinated green beans, good olives, and herb dressing

1:00 PM	**SELF-TLC**
	Option: Create a Week Two vision board (collage) of your goals or add to one that you may have started in Week One
	Option: Contemplate today's action step for Aligning with Your Ultimate Purpose

DAY **8** ★

4:00 PM   DINNER

Recipe of the Day: Green Noodles (page 308)

6:00 PM   GET YOUR GLOW ON

Put your legs up the wall and listen to music or read for fifteen minutes

---

AS DESIRED   SNACKS & DESSERTS

1 piece of fruit

Sheets of seaweed (nori)

7:00 PM   DUSK GLOW TONIC

Cooling water with the juice of half a lemon and slices of orange and cucumber

---

SUPPLEMENTAL RECOMMENDATION

Take one to three enzymes (as suggested according to brand) with each meal to aid digestion and cellular cleansing.

DAY EIGHT **TOOLKIT**

Virtue of the Day: *Reverence*

Reverence is both a feeling and an attitude of deep respect, transformational as a state of devotional love. Although we often think of reverence in relationship to great teachers and spiritual leaders, it is also an energy that we can bring to virtually anyone or any moment. The twenty-one-day journey you have committed to is an act of reverence you are extending to yourself. Allow that thought to permeate your awareness today as you honor your divine nature and bow to the beauty of the physical body and all it makes possible.

Action Step of the Day: *Aligning with Your Ultimate Purpose*

Now is the time to feel good about what you're putting into your body and *on* your body. When we think of cleansing and avoiding toxins, very few of us would think about the clothing we wear. But did you know that the number one genetically modified crop in the entire world is cotton? Also, have you ever tried to walk around in one of those polyester jerseys, much less work out in them? If you are not already doing this, consider sourcing your clothing from sustainable and organic companies; this is another tangible way for you to care for the earth while caring for yourself too.

RECIPE OF THE DAY: **GREEN NOODLES**

A power-packed live food feast for beauty and nutritional replenishment.

INGREDIENTS

- 1 package kelp noodles or 3 zucchini (cut in spirals)
- 1 cup soaked almonds
- 2 cups kale
- 1 heirloom tomato
- ½ cup red bell pepper
- ½ avocado
- 1 tablespoon olive oil
- ½ tablespoon Bragg Liquid Aminos (or nama shoyu or tamari)
- ½ tablespoon lemon juice
- 2 cloves garlic
- Cayenne pepper to taste

DIRECTIONS

1. Add everything except the noodles of choice to the blender and blend.
2. Add the blended dressing on top of the noodles and enjoy!
3. Option: If you have one, warm in the dehydrator for a couple of hours or until warm and soft.

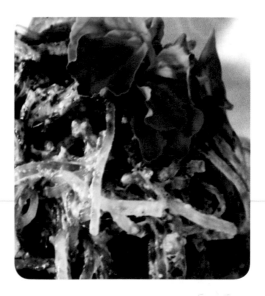

DAY EIGHT **TOOLKIT**

Yoga Pose of the Day: *Lion Pose*

Kneel on the floor, sitting back onto your heels. Press your palms firmly against your knees. Fan your palms and splay your fingers like the razor-sharp claws of a large feline. Breathe deeply, inhaling through your nose. As you prepare to exhale, simultaneously open your mouth wide, stretching your tongue out while curling

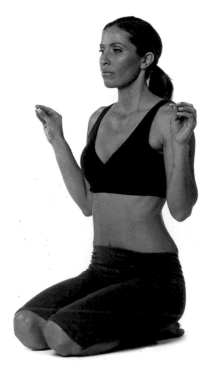

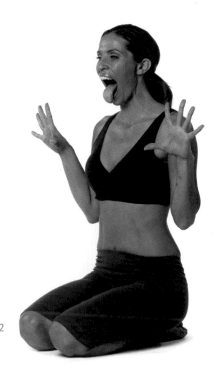

1

2

DAY **8**

its tip down toward your chin. Stretch wide and exhale with force, breathing out through your mouth with a hissing "ha" sound or even a loud roar. Breathing normally, release the tensions that may be affecting your posture and your jaw, and potentially creating wrinkles. Repeat this cycle; I like to do it six times.

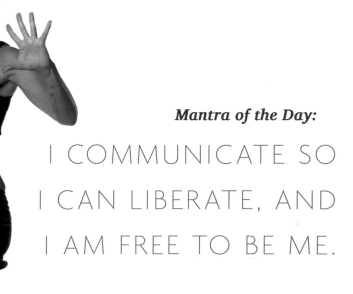

3

Mantra of the Day:

I COMMUNICATE SO I CAN LIBERATE, AND I AM FREE TO BE ME.

DAY NINE **SCHEDULE**

7:00 AM   DAWN GLOW TONIC
Hot Apple Cider Tea (page 334)
Option: Liver Kick (page 94)

8:00 AM   BREAKFAST
Flax crackers or live food bread with coconut oil and cinnamon
Option: a superfood smoothie

10:00 AM   YOGA POSE OF THE DAY
Option: *Yoga for Beauty* Pose of the Day
Option: Try a dance class or turn your living room into a
dance studio for thirty minutes!

12:00 NOON   LUNCH
Recipe of the Day: Live Spring Rolls (page 309)
Cup of green tea with lemon and raw honey or decaffeinated
chai with live almond milk.

1:00 PM   SELF-TLC
Option: Read an inspiring book passage
Option: Contemplate today's action step for Aligning with
Your Ultimate Purpose

DAY **9** ★

4:00 PM	DINNER
	Morning Miso Soup (page 316); create your own version of the recipe by adding ingredients such as leeks, chives, thyme, shredded nori, carrots, moringa powder, or something else that lights you up

6:00 PM	GET YOUR GLOW ON
	Treat yourself to a luxurious Beauty Bath. See the Superstar Skin section on page 274 to find your head-to-toe glow.

AS DESIRED	SNACKS & DESSERTS
	1 piece of fruit
	3 dates with almond butter

7:00 PM	DUSK GLOW TONIC
	Blessed Delight Tea (page 331)

SUPPLEMENTAL RECOMMENDATIONS

Support your cleanse with two capsules of charcoal a day to bind and remove toxins. (All supplements can be done throughout the program.)

DAY NINE **TOOLKIT**

Virtue of the Day: *Charity*

Sometimes we greedily cling to things that no longer add to the quality of our lives—whether those "things" are material possessions, habits, attitudes, behaviors, or certain foods—because we're afraid that without them, important needs will not get met. This very human concern is an invitation to approach ourselves with charity. What that can mean on this ninth day of your cleansing journey is taking a moment to look within. What do you need right now? How can you be lusciously generous with yourself? Do you need to ask for support of some kind? Will you let others offer their assistance to you? As we let ourselves receive, our ability to give is amplified. Also, when we open ourselves to giving to others, we are also opening ourselves to receiving.

Action Step of the Day: *Aligning with Your Ultimate Purpose*

Try a new food today. Venture into the grocery store or stroll along the farmers market stands looking to see what foods draw your attention, especially in the abundant world of fruits and vegetables. Is there an exotic fruit, a type of leafy green, or even a delectable raw goody that seems to pique your curiosity and say, "Pick me!"? Taking it to the next level: once you find a food you've never tried before, imagine a new use for it. By trying new things, you are potentially opening yourself up to new flavors, textures, and aromas, as well as new combinations of vitamins, minerals, and other phytonutrients. Exploring new foods might also be the precursor to trying other new things—from experiences to thoughts and feelings.

RECIPE OF THE DAY: **LIVE SPRING ROLLS**

An Asian-influenced meal that is easy to make and bursting with flavor and crunch.

INGREDIENTS—ROLL FILLING:

- ½ bunch collard greens
- 2 to 3 carrots, julienned
- ¼ head purple cabbage, shredded
- ¾ cup minced almonds

INGREDIENTS—SAUCE:

- ¼ cup onions, mashed (to release flavor)
- 2 tablespoons nama shoyu
- 2 tablespoons sweetener (maple syrup is great in this, and although not live, it's mineral rich)
- 1 teaspoon toasted sesame oil, or chopped almonds as an alternative
- ½ juiced orange

DIRECTIONS

1. Wash the collard green leaves and remove the hard stems.
2. Toss all the chopped vegetables in half the sauce for a more decadent option, or simply keep to the side for dipping.
3. Fill the leaves with the carrots, cabbage, almonds, and anything else you would like to put inside.
4. Roll the leaves into spring roll shapes to contain the filling.
5. Mix the sauce ingredients together in a separate bowl.
6. Dip the rolls in the remainder of the sauce. Enjoy!

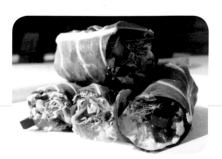

DAY NINE TOOLKIT

Yoga for Beauty Pose of the Day: *Seated Hip Opener*

Begin in Staff Pose *(Dandasana),* legs out in front and back straight and strong. Lift your chest. Let your shoulders slide away from your ears. Bend your right knee and place your right ankle and flexed foot just above the left kneecap. Move the knee away from your body to begin to open the hip. Keep your back straight as you bring your right leg up toward your chest. Stay for at least five long breaths and then repeat on the second side.

Mantra of the Day:

I AM SUPPORTED AND GROUNDED, FROM WHERE I'M FOUNDED.

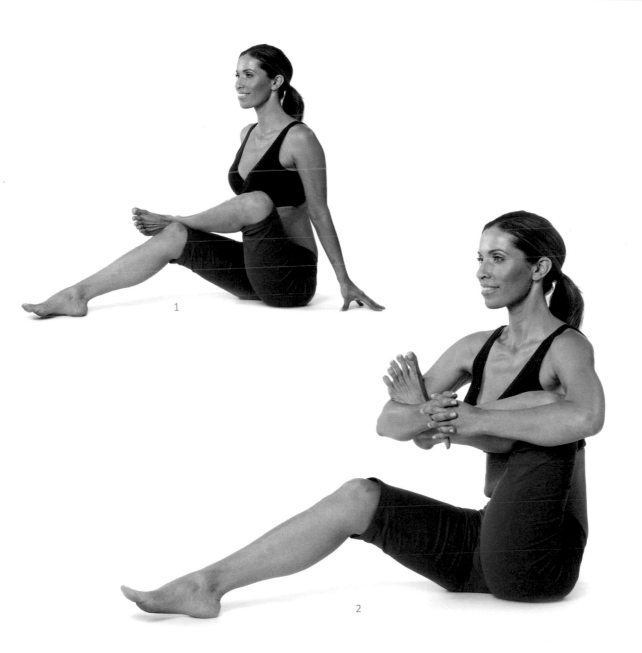

1

2

DAY TEN **SCHEDULE**

7:00 AM   DAWN GLOW TONIC
1 cup of hot water with lemon or other liver tonic of your choice

8:00 AM   BREAKFAST
½ mini-watermelon, cut in half; eat with a spoon
1 cup of hot yerba maté (choosing tea bags at this point)
Option: Live Chocolate Shake (page 334)

10:00 AM   YOGA POSE OF THE DAY
Option: *Yoga for Beauty* Pose of the Day
Option: And/or try a local yoga class (make it a super-yoga day)

12:00 NOON   LUNCH
Recipe of the Day: Kale & Avocado Salad (page 319)
Plus … Rainbeau's Guilt-Free Strawberry Pie (page 328)

1:00 PM   SELF-TLC
Option: Spend some quiet time in a steambath or sauna (at the Y?)
Option: Contemplate today's action step for Aligning with
Your Ultimate Purpose

DAY **10** ★

4:00 PM   DINNER

Chop cabbage in the food processor and massage with lemon, olive oil, Celtic sea salt, and a touch of raw honey; add avocado slices, chopped almonds, or shredded seaweed and/or dill

6:00 PM   GET YOUR GLOW ON

Swim at the beach or in a pool (preferably non-chlorinated)

AS DESIRED   SNACKS & DESSERTS

1 flax cracker or other raw-ingredient cracker or bread with a touch of raw honey

7:00 PM   DUSK GLOW TONIC

Lemonade with maple syrup and hint of cayenne

SUPPLEMENTAL RECOMMENDATION

As you eat these foods that are bursting with life, envision that you are lighting up each cell of your body with the vital nutrients it needs for glowing health.

DAY TEN **TOOLKIT**

Virtue of the Day: *Empathy*

You are halfway through this week of activating your body and mind with live foods, whether you have chosen to eat only living foods or have greatly increased the percentage of living foods while remaining 100 percent vegan. How has this sensitized you to your inner world and the world around you? Do you feel more empathy with others, identifying more intimately with their feelings and thoughts while maintaining your own boundaries? At the heart of it, empathy is a soulful responsiveness to others, a way of being in community with the world around us. As you proceed through this day, notice how the warmth of your own understanding is a gift to those around you.

Action Step of the Day: *Aligning with Your Ultimate Purpose*

Grow a new habit today, literally. Be a kitchen gardener today and sprout some buckwheat, sunflower seeds, or other desired sprouts. Not only are the sprouts some of the most nutritious foods you can eat (and satisfying in their crunchy deliciousness), but the greater gift is the fulfillment of bringing something new into your life and into this world. See the Sprouting Guide on page 359 in Rainbeau's Reading Room.

RECIPE OF THE DAY: **KALE & AVOCADO SALAD**

Enjoy the superior nutritional profile of this hearty and flavorful salad.

INGREDIENTS

- ½ bunch kale
- 1 ripe avocado
- ¼ onion, chopped
- ¼ cup shredded purple cabbage
- ¼ cup olive oil
- ½ lemon, juiced
- ½ teaspoon nama shoyu
- 1 tablespoon sweetener of choice (raw honey, agave, etc.)
- Sesame seeds for garnish

DIRECTIONS

1. Break the kale into bite-sized pieces; chop the avocado into small pieces.
2. Combine the kale, avocado, onions, and purple cabbage into one bowl.
3. Mix the olive oil, lemon juice, nama shoyu, and sweetener together in a separate bowl to create a dressing/marinade for the salad.
4. Use clean hands to massage the marinade into the kale and all the other veggies until soft.
5. Let the salad marinate for about an hour, then enjoy!
6. Option: If you have leftovers, you can dehydrate and make delicious veggie chips by simply spreading the mixture onto a dehydrator tray.

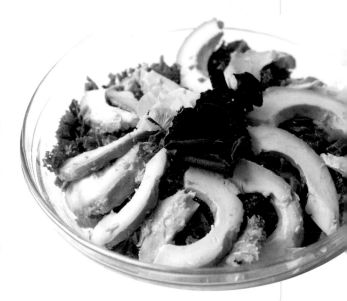

DAY TEN **TOOLKIT**

Yoga for Beauty Pose of the Day: *Wind-Relieving Pose*

This posture, *Pavanamuktasana* in Sanskrit, improves digestion and elimination while stretching the low back and lengthening the spine. Lie relaxed on your back and pull both legs in toward your core. Grasp your hands around your knees to gently pull your legs closer into the sides of the chest. Remain in this posture for seven breath cycles or for as long as is comfortable. Massage the internal organs to promote detoxification, and on each exhale draw the legs closer into the body that is home to all the vital organs of elimination. Deep breathing assists with the flow of nourishing blood and oxygen to these areas. After seven breath cycles, release your arms and legs back down to the floor and feel, lengthening down through your sit bones and widening the back of your body as you support your organs and open the hips.

DAY 10

Mantra of the Day:

It hurts too much to look inside but God you already see and you've forgiven me and healed me & I don't have to walk ashamed any more I release my demands & failures & I open myself up for total wholeness that others will be touched because you have set me free

I BEGIN WHERE I AM AND ACCEPT MYSELF.

I HAVE NOWHERE TO GO BUT WITHIN.

171

DAY ELEVEN SCHEDULE

7:00 AM   DAWN GLOW TONIC
Start with liver tonic of your choice
Yerba Maté Latte (page 337)

8:00 AM   BREAKFAST
1 bowl of soaked chia with the additions you like (such as fruit, cacao nibs, or coconut flakes)
1 cup of hot herbal tea
Option: Papaya, cinnamon, and raw honey smoothie

10:00 AM   YOGA POSE OF THE DAY
Option: *Yoga for Beauty* Pose of the Day
Option: Try a local Tai Chi or martial arts class

12:00 NOON   LUNCH
Recipe of the Day: Celery Chowder (page 315)

1:00 PM   SELF-TLC
Option: Practice conscious breathing (*pranayama*)
Option: Contemplate today's action step for Aligning with Your Ultimate Purpose

DAY 11 ★

4:00 PM	DINNER

Improv Pizza: Take the raw pizza crust, flax crackers, or other type of raw crackers you may have on hand and spread on a generous amount of Herb Pesto (recipe page 322) or tomato sauce. Then top with sliced tomato, olives, sun-dried tomatoes, veggies, a bit of chili powder, and a sprinkle of nutritional yeast.

6:00 PM	GET YOUR GLOW ON

Play! Turn on upbeat music and just dance!

AS DESIRED	SNACKS & DESSERTS

Jicama Fries (page 322) or sliced jicama chips with Guacamole (page 321) or other raw dip of choice.
Fun tip: for guacamole with a twist, add a hint of Cajun spice.

7:00 PM	DUSK GLOW TONIC

Fresh coconut water or Divine Organics coconut water in glass bottle

SUPPLEMENTAL RECOMMENDATION

Write down what you're craving at this point in your all-living-foods journey. See how the act of jotting your cravings onto paper might alter them (take out your journal or just write a simple list). While you're at it, enjoy one handful of a superfood trail mix, like cacao nibs, macadamia nuts, and golden berries. What fun—to write about cravings while eating a supernutrition treat!

DAY ELEVEN TOOLKIT

Virtue of the Day: *Wholeheartedness*

When we embark on any kind of transformational journey, we are inevitably confronted with aspects of ourselves that resist change, that are comfortable with things staying just as they are. Over the previous ten days, have you noticed any resistance to change within yourself? Sometimes this inner friction disguises itself as fatigue, exhaustion, or what can look like outright laziness. Although a nap and green juice wouldn't hurt, the deeper solution is to put your attention on something that engages your whole heart. That is what wholeheartedness really is—an unequivocal "yes!" that tells you when you're in alignment with the person you are becoming. Take some time today, whether five minutes or a few hours, when you actively focus your attention on something that has your whole heart. As the saying goes, "Either do something with your whole heart or don't do it at all."

Action Step of the Day: *Aligning with Your Ultimate Purpose*

Today is an opportunity to literally align yourself, focusing on decompressing your spine. Our day-to-day activities—especially all our sitting in chairs, cars, and couches—can take a toll on our bodies by impacting the spine. To counter this, simple forward folds can help release tension in the body. Also, hanging from a stable bar (like monkey bars on the playground) will help alleviate tension from top to bottom. Plus it gives you a good excuse to visit a nearby park. Once you find your bar to hang from, spend at least ten full breaths in this playful posture.

DAY 11

RECIPE OF THE DAY: **CELERY CHOWDER**

With garlic and cayenne adding the heat, this soup recipe is warming and awakening.

INGREDIENTS

- 1 cup macadamia nuts
- 7 to 8 stalks celery: 5 to 6 chopped for blending and 2 to 3 diced
- 2 chopped squash
- 2 cloves garlic
- ½ avocado
- Pinch Celtic sea salt
- Cayenne to taste
- 1 sprig rosemary or to taste
- 1 teaspoon extra virgin olive oil

DIRECTIONS

1. Combine all the ingredients except the diced celery into a blender with enough water to completely cover everything.
2. Blend everything until smooth and creamy. Add water to change the consistency.
3. Stir the diced celery into the soup for extra texture.
4. Add a few slices of avocado on top and drizzle on some olive oil for a final touch.

You can heat this soup on the stove to slightly warm it up if you desire, taking care not to warm it up to the point where it would no longer be considered raw.

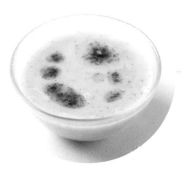

DAY ELEVEN TOOLKIT

Yoga for Beauty Pose of the Day: *Deep Squat*

Begin by standing with your feet shoulder-width apart and your toes point-ing slightly outward. Reach your arms overhead to elongate your spine, then slowly lower into a squat (Chair Pose), consciously keeping your spine as straight as possible. Beginners should simply come down first without the extra core challenge of holding your arms up. If this position is challenging, remain here for a few breaths and return to standing. Alternatively, to deepen the posture, sink fully into a deep squat, resting your upper arms on your knees and grounding through the feet. In the full pose, the soles of your feet will remain on the floor, but if necessary slide down a wall for support and balance, put a chair in front of you to hold onto, or put a blanket underneath your heels. Be mindful not to push past your present limits, going only as deep into your squat as is comfortable. Surrender to gravity as you breathe deeply for several cycles. After five to ten breaths, press your feet into the floor as you come back into standing position. Shake your legs out to release any ten-sion. Wherever you have cultivated a feeling of warmth in your body, visual-ize red light permeating down through those areas—then draw that warm, red energy upward to maintain the sensation of grounding throughout the whole body. For deeper results, try adding in the *ra'yoKa* squat sequence we do in our Level Red practice (available in *ra'yoKa* downloads).

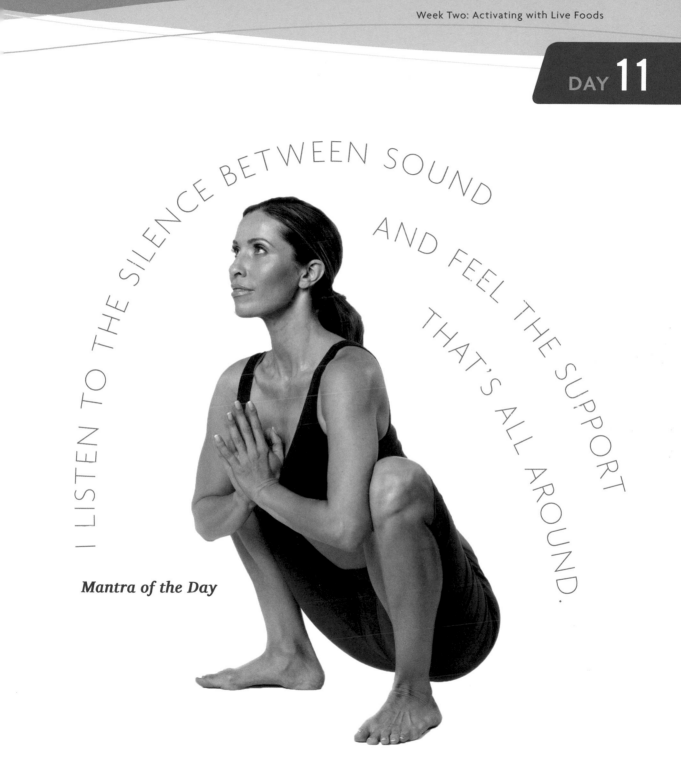

I LISTEN TO THE SILENCE BETWEEN SOUND AND FEEL THE SUPPORT THAT'S ALL AROUND.

Mantra of the Day

DAY TWELVE SCHEDULE

7:00 AM DAWN GLOW TONIC
Start with the liver tonic of your choice
Follow with a tea of holy basil, lemon, and raw honey for a
day of euphoria *Note: holy basil is also known as tulsi*

8:00 AM BREAKFAST
Jumpstart Chia Breakfast (page 325)
Yerba maté (just a bag; try adding ginger and mint for
support)
Option: Strawberry and cream smoothie—blend strawberries,
fresh almond milk, raw honey, a pinch of Celtic sea salt, and
a touch of fresh vanilla

10:00 AM YOGA POSE OF THE DAY
Option: *Yoga for Beauty* Pose of the Day
Option: Try a *ra'yoKa* from the DVD or download

12:00 NOON LUNCH
Have an amazing Mediterranean salad with everything raw:
mixed greens, sun-dried tomatoes, crumbled Nut Cheese
(page 323), plus hearty additions such as chopped and
marinated green beans, good olives, and an herb dressing

DAY 12 ★

1:00 PM   SELF-TLC

Option: Take an afternoon bubble bath

Option: Contemplate today's action step for Aligning with Your Ultimate Purpose

4:00 PM   DINNER

Recipe of the Day: Raw Popcorn (page 323)

Plus … Quick Raw Tomato Soup (page 317)

6:00 PM   GET YOUR GLOW ON

Option: Unleash your energy—go for a run, walk, or jog

AS DESIRED   SNACKS & DESSERTS

Leftover Guilt-Free Strawberry Pie

Easy Breezy Smoothie: take all the ingredients within a coconut and blend with vanilla and coconut oil—yum!

7:00 PM   DUSK GLOW TONIC

Blend fresh almond milk with a teaspoon of cacao and some raw honey. Who says you can't have chocolate milk? Enjoy!

SUPPLEMENTAL RECOMMENDATIONS

Think of adding psyllium seed husks to your diet to clean out the small intestine, but do not overdo this. Gentle is the way.

DAY TWELVE **TOOLKIT**

Virtue of the Day: *Honesty*

In addition to fruits, vegetables, water, and exercise, honesty itself is one of the most potent detoxifiers and healers available to us. Honesty was likely involved in your decision to find your SuperStar Cleanse in the first place—as you truthfully acknowledged that there is something you want and need, with extraordinary health being a part of that equation. Today, celebrate the honesty that put you on this path of healthful eating and regeneration. Engaging fully in this twenty-one-day cleanse is an act of loving self-responsibility that can skyrocket your confidence, opening doors that you may not have imagined before now.

Action Step of the Day: *Aligning with Your Ultimate Purpose*

What are you sleeping on? Our environment, air, and food are all important, but how about where we spend a third of our lives … *in our beds!* Yes, it's been said that regular commercial mattresses can be hosts for dust mites and chemicals, so if you still need to save for that organic (non-spring) bed and organic pillows, consider using dust mite covers for your bed and pillows. Place all your bedding and pillows in the dryer for forty-five minutes once a month. Spray lavender or eucalyptus on washed sheets. Make sure you're washing at least your bedding (if not all your laundry) in environmentally friendly laundry soap. Try sleeping on your back for enhanced face care and using a fancy fit-to-your-neck pillow. Also consider being lower to the ground or at least sleeping without anything below you (clear the clutter from beneath your bed). Sleep deep, be merry, and write down your dreams for greater understanding of what they are conveying to you.

RECIPE OF THE DAY: **RAW POPCORN**

This easy recipe is proof that living foods are fun! The popcorn does not have to be dehydrated to be enjoyed and often is eaten before the job is done anyway.

INGREDIENTS

- 1 head cauliflower
- ½ cup nutritional yeast
- ¼ cup olive oil
- Pinch of Celtic sea salt

DIRECTIONS

1. Chop the cauliflower florets into small popcorn-sized bits and put them in a bowl.

2. Add the nutritional yeast, salt, and oil to the bowl and cover the cauliflower completely with the mixture.

3. Option: You can dehydrate the cauliflower for up to 4 hours or longer for a more distinct popcorn texture and taste.

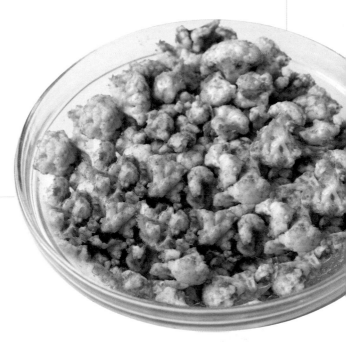

DAY TWELVE TOOLKIT

Yoga for Beauty Pose of the Day: *Half Frog Pose*

Begin by lying on your belly and press your forearms into the floor while lifting your upper torso and head. Bend both knees out to the sides and allow your feet to extend back behind you. Hips anchor down as you round the back and shift back toward your feet. Ground down and push back, breathing into whatever you may have been sitting on that is congesting your hips, thighs, and groin. Stay here for about five minutes, eyes closed and mind still—cry if you need to. Release, come back, and pause in Child's Pose. Let the grace of your body's full breath move you into, through, and out of this posture.

Important: It is possible that this pose could be highly uncomfortable and even bring you to the edge of what you might call pain. If it's too much, start with only one leg at a time, and notice the difference between sharp pain (which is cautionary) and the discomfort of deep, thick, old stuff being stored that must be faced in order to move. I must admit that this is my least easy pose, so I re-label it my favorite and breathe.

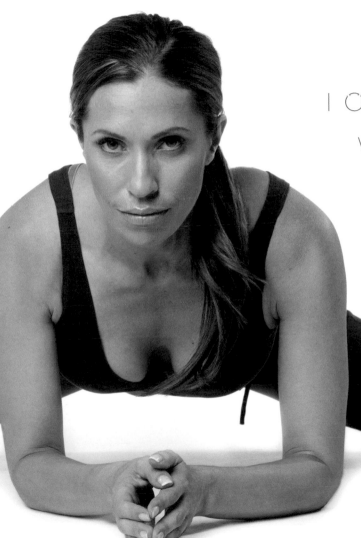

Mantra of the Day:

I OPEN AND ALIGN
WITH GUIDANCE
THAT'S DIVINE,
I AM ONE WITH
THE HIGHEST
HIGH.

DAY THIRTEEN SCHEDULE

7:00 AM   DAWN GLOW TONIC
Liver Kick (page 94)
Yerba maté (one optional bag) with nettles and red
raspberry leaf

8:00 AM   BREAKFAST
Chia Pudding (page 326)—spice it up however you like

10:00 AM   YOGA POSE OF THE DAY
Option: *Yoga for Beauty* Pose of the Day
Option: Shoot some hoops at a local court

12:00 NOON   LUNCH
Nori wrap containing smashed avocado with Celtic sea salt
and cumin—simple but so satisfying. Kids like it simple; even
my daughter goes for this one. Think about adding tomatoes
and sunflower sprouts.

1:00 PM   SELF-TLC
Option: Listen to a guided meditation or visualization
Option: Contemplate today's action step for Aligning with
Your Ultimate Purpose

4:00 PM	DINNER
	Recipe of the Day: Cheesy Vegetable Medley (page 306)

6:00 PM	GET YOUR GLOW ON
	Try a local Tai Chi or art class

AS DESIRED	SNACKS & DESSERTS
	Chocolate Mousse-Dipped Strawberries (page 327)
	Option: Moringa Bliss Balls (page 328)

7:00 PM	DUSK GLOW TONIC
	Green Clean Juice (page 333)

SUPPLEMENTAL RECOMMENDATION

Get to know and love your nettles! Drink nettles tea every day for blood, bone, and kidney support. My favorite herb, as well as my mom's, this one can be used internally or fresh topically for arthritis, cellulite, hair loss, or wrinkles. A miracle plant!

DAY THIRTEEN **TOOLKIT**

Virtue of the Day: *Self-Control*

The dark side of living in a world where we have an abundance of choices, from the many sinful temptations to food that is made up of chemicals, is that giving in to instant gratification can and most likely will lead to the proverbial "vicious cycle." This is especially true when we put things into our minds or systems that are opposite of the intentions that our beings are striving for. The more we take in, the less we are nourished—and the cravings and habits continue and strengthen. As we near the end of Week Two, if you find yourself distracted or even consumed by addiction, make a decision to invoke self-control. Call on the inner strength that comes from an awareness that you have a purpose to fulfill on this planet and are worthy of exquisite, lifelong well-being.

Action Step of the Day: *Aligning with Your Ultimate Purpose*

Cultivate gratitude for all the support you have. As you engage in this journey of healthy eating, ask a true friend for their support, and then acknowledge that support when it comes. While it may not always be easy to integrate your food choices with theirs, here are some tips to help bring healthy foods successfully into your home.

- Let your friend know that you are not expecting them to join you in your new diet, but you look forward to having more raw foods available at meals so that you can enjoy eating together.
- Slowly increase the amount of raw food on the table.
- Enjoy a well-dressed and satisfying salad before indulging in the cooked meal so your enzymes are supporting your digestion.

RECIPE OF THE DAY: **CHEESY VEGETABLE MEDLEY**

This nutritiously filling dish is the perfect marriage of crunchy and creamy.

INGREDIENTS—VEGETABLE MEDLEY

- 1 baby bok choy
- ½ cauliflower
- 2 carrots
- 2 zucchini
- 1 cup olive oil
- Celtic sea salt

INGREDIENTS—NUT CHEESE

- 1 cup macadamia or other raw nut
- 1 tablespoon lemon juice
- 2 garlic cloves
- 2 tablespoons olive oil
- Coriander to taste
- Curry to taste
- Chili pepper to taste

DIRECTIONS

1. Cut up the vegetables and marinate in olive oil and salt.
2. While the vegetables are marinating, blend the ingredients for nut cheese.
3. Cover the vegetables with the nut cheese and mix well.
4. Dehydrate the mixture until the vegetables are softened (about 4 hours).

Note: Although this dish is better prepared in the dehydrator, if you don't have one, there are options. You can put it in a window in the hot sun or outside in the sun (covered with a screen to protect from bugs). A friend of mine used a thermometer to check the heat of her stove while warmed only by the pilot light, and it was 115° F exactly—where there is a will, there is a way. Regarding dehydrators, you can buy them inexpensively nowadays, so consider making the investment for your health … and for the pleasure of your taste buds.

DAY THIRTEEN **TOOLKIT**

- Find out what kind of foods friends and family members enjoy, and make raw versions of those dishes.
- Most important, let go of the need to change others. You will impress people more with your health and vitality than you ever will with preaching. Be a living example of what you represent.

Yoga for Beauty Pose of the Day: *Supported Legs up the Wall or Block Pose*

This posture is a gentle and restorative inversion that keeps the hips slightly elevated, allowing gravity to assist blood flow from the extremities to the vital organs, heart, and head. Utilize this posture frequently to aid digestion and calm the mind.

For your support, you will need either a block or one to two thickly folded blankets. You'll also need a place where you can comfortably rest your legs vertically (or nearly so) on a wall or other upright support. If you are tall or tend to be stiff, you will want to position blankets lower and farther from the wall. If you are shorter and/or flexible, use a higher support and position yourself closer to the wall. The wall is not necessary when using a block, so adjust the instructions accordingly.

Sit sideways on the floor beside the wall, knees bent, with one shoulder and hip touching the wall. As you lower your back to the floor, exhale. With one smooth movement, swing your legs up onto the wall and your shoulders and head lightly down onto the floor. Release and elongate through the back of your neck and soften your throat. Allow your shoulder blades to open wide away from the spine, and splay your hands and arms out to your sides, keeping palms facing up. Your legs should be held somewhat firmly to keep them vertically in place against the wall while sinking the weight of your hips and belly as they soften in to the floor. Breathe deeply for five to fifteen minutes.

When complete, slide off the support onto the floor before turning to the side and coming back to a seated position. *Note: Do not turn your head in this pose.*

Mantra of the Day: PEACE BEGINS WITHIN ME AND CONTINUES ON INTO THE WORLD.

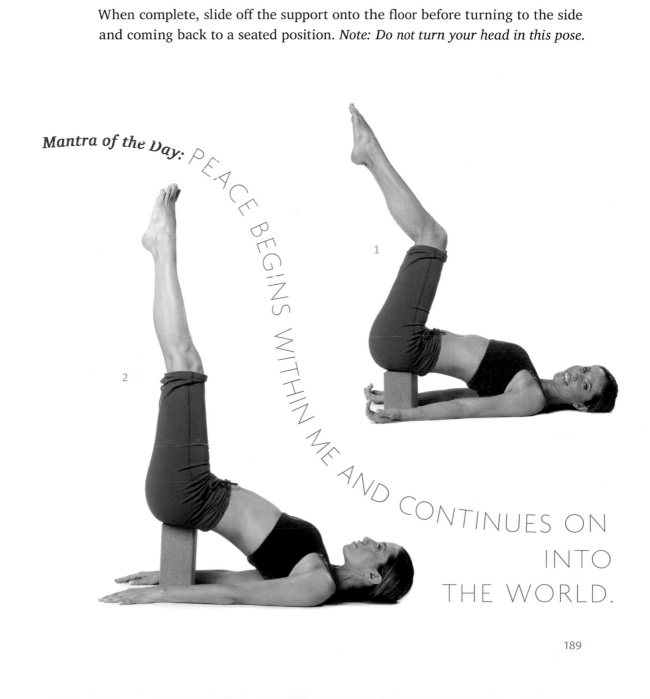

DAY FOURTEEN **SCHEDULE**

7:00 AM   DAWN GLOW TONIC

Start with the liver tonic of your choice

Hot Apple Cider Tea (page 334)

8:00AM   BREAKFAST

Chia Pudding (page 326)—garnish with whatever your heart desires, as long as it's raw

10:00 AM   YOGA POSE OF THE DAY

Option: *Yoga for Beauty* Pose of the Day

Option: Time to get your groove on again. Turn on upbeat music and dance! (Clothes are optional.)

12:00 NOON   LUNCH

Recipe of the Day: Rainbeau's Favorite Herb Salad (page 320)

1:00 PM   SELF-TLC

Option: Journal about what you've experienced so far

Option: Contemplate today's action step for Aligning with Your Ultimate Purpose

| 4:00 PM | DINNER |
| | Chopped and marinated vegetables. Simply blend unpasteurized miso with water and add veggies of your choice. Sprinkle with chopped chives and enjoy with an avocado and tomato capresc salad |

| 6:00 PM | GET YOUR GLOW ON |
| | Try *Yoga for Beauty: Dusk* DVD to help wind down for the night |

| AS DESIRED | SNACKS & DESSERTS |
| | Try some type of fruit you have never tried before. Have you explored the flavors of dragon fruit or pineapple guava? |

| 7:00 PM | DUSK GLOW TONIC |
| | Peppermint tea with raw honey and lemon |

SUPPLEMENTAL RECOMMENDATION

Today the theme is herbs. Consider ingesting some herbs with each meal, whether fresh or dried. While thcy are incredibly delicious, herbs are also rich in vitamins, phytonutrients, and essential oils that offer many benefits, including being antibacterial and supportive to the immune system.

DAY FOURTEEN **TOOLKIT**

Virtue of the Day: *Patience*

Having arrived at Day Fourteen, two-thirds of the way to health transformation, you have likely experienced a wide range of emotions … and not all comfortable ones! It is so important during a cleanse to be reminded that challenging thoughts and feelings often come to the surface—*and this is a good thing.* When feelings such as irritation, restlessness, and anger emerge, it is often a sign that old toxins are being released from the body and mind. Paradoxically, being patient with yourself when minor or major annoyances arise will help you weather the little storms. Today, look for an oasis of inner calm. This is where you can dip your toes into the pool of patience that reflects back to you the persistent courage that brought you to this moment. When in doubt, place your hands on your heart and ask to return there.

Action Step of the Day: *Aligning with Your Ultimate Purpose*

Get more sunlight! The sun is the source of all life on this planet. Did you know there are millions of receptors in the eyes that turn sunlight into vitamins? The sun ignites protons to heat up and bring toxins and poisons to the largest organ of the body: the skin. During your cleanse, that is especially important, as the skin is able to release the toxins that you are committed to flushing out of your system. Studies have also shown that being exposed to sunlight improves our mood, helping alleviate symptoms of depression. Although there are variances in how much sunlight is needed each day, in general ten to thirty minutes a day of unfiltered sunlight (including no sunscreen) will positively affect your body and spirit. Allowing yourself to be kissed by the sun will help you look upon the world with clarity and optimism, not to mention provide you with your vital vitamin D.

DAY 14

RECIPE OF THE DAY: **RAINBEAU'S FAVORITE HERB SALAD**

So simple, delicious, aromatic, and healing … I make this salad all the time now and eat it as a main dish, although it also makes a beautiful garnish for any meal.

INGREDIENTS

- 1 bunch of fresh parsley
- 1 bunch of fresh mint
- 1 bunch of fresh basil
- 1 bunch of cilantro (optional)
- 1 bunch of fresh dill
- 1 lemon
- ¼ cup extra virgin olive oil, to taste
- Celtic sea salt, to taste

DIRECTIONS

1. De-stem all these amazing plants and then start chopping. *Note: If you can, use a ceramic knife, as it keeps these herbs from turning brown.*
2. Toss into a bowl together and add in a liberal amount of olive oil, lemon, and Celtic sea salt. Herbs tend to absorb quickly, so depending on the amount of fresh herbs you're using, modify these flavor-enhancing and preserving condiments.

Goodness … even as I write I wish I had some ready to eat. This lively salad makes you feel clean and refreshed from the inside out.

DAY FOURTEEN TOOLKIT

Yoga for Beauty Pose of the Day: *Tree Pose*

This is called *Vrksasana* in Sanskrit (*vrksa* means tree). How does a tree grow flowers and fruits? By rooting deep into the ground. Begin by standing in *tadasana,* Mountain Pose. Shift your weight onto the left foot, rooting through the inner foot into the floor. While gently bending your right knee, reach down and clasp your right ankle, placing the sole of your right foot against the inner left thigh, toes pointing toward the floor (option for advanced practitioners: press your right heel into the inner left groin, toes pointing toward the floor). Keeping the center of your pelvis directly over the left foot, lengthen your tailbone toward the floor and extend your arms up. Like the tree, connect to the complementary energetic forces and support provided by gravity (ground through your roots for your foundation) and find loftiness (elevating your branches to blossom your fruits toward the sun). Practice each side for at least ten full breaths. Step back into Mountain Pose with an exhalation and repeat on the other side. Use a wall or chair for additional balance if needed.

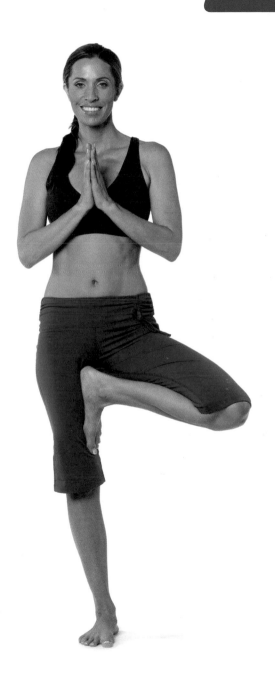

Mantra of the Day:

I AM

THE TREE.

EVERYTHING

I NEED IS

WITHIN

ME.

ILLUMINATIONS
week two

With a cup of tea or superfood smoothie in hand, enjoy the following section, designed to deepen your understanding of the cleanse process and expand your level of inspiration.

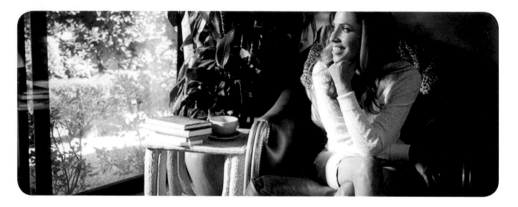

The Abundance of Living Foods: *Tips for Succeeding in the Living*

Eating living foods is all about feeling happy, joyous, and *alive!* This is your week for further shifting your thinking to an attitude of abundance. Remember: you can eat anything you want as long as it is living and helps you thrive. Eat as many fresh veggies, greens, fruits, and healthy fats as possible—flaxseeds, chia seeds, coconuts, avocado, sprouted grains, and soaked seeds and nuts. The marinades you use and the spices you choose will make it all the more enjoyable.

We will continue the practice of starting each day with a liver tonic (choose the one that calls to you on any given day, whether it's the Liver Kick one day, the ACV Tonic another, or simply a cup of warm water with half a squeezed lemon). Then, approximately twenty to forty minutes after the morning drink, have a smoothie or chocolate shake (preferably with raw cacao powder or nibs and some maca). Exciting!

While we transition to living foods this week, we'll begin to incorporate more of the blended foods that will be our focus in Week Three. Not only is blending an easy way to get living foods into your body with less stress; it renders outrageously delicious concoctions! In addition to chocolate shakes and berry smoothies, we'll begin to add blended soups (like gazpacho) into our meal plans, as well as heartier dishes like raw tacos and wraps, seed cheeses, raw sandwiches, and blended desserts made with coconut and other fruits.

The following tips and suggestions are offered to make Week Two not only successful but pleasurable too:

Prepare ahead with shopping, soaking, chopping, and all other food preparation. It's not the same as grabbing something last-minute at a deli, but it is so worth the extra time and attention. It's also a way to ensure that you put yourself at the top of your daily priority list.

About shopping: know what you need before you make a trip to the grocery store. You don't want to get home and realize you forgot something for your recipes and creations (no need for this kind of frustration or discouragement). Using the recommended shopping list as your guide, do your best to prepare a list of necessary and desired items ahead of time.

Choose organic, go for a wide variety of colors, and get to know and love the produce and bulk sections of your favorite store.

Try every farmers market at your disposal—this is where you get the freshest produce at the best prices.

When using greens like kale, you will want to break down the plant fibers by massaging the greens with lemon, olive oil, and salt to make them more digestible. This is a mainstay for my family, and it's always a hit!

Soak and rinse your nuts and seeds to remove enzyme inhibitors. This is the magic key to making them more digestible—with the added bonus of making them easier to use for creamy dishes like seed cheeses and smooth desserts.

Have fun incorporating superfoods into your smoothies, desserts, and other compatible recipes. Maca, cacao, acai, and lucuma are four highly beneficial and tasty options.

When eating out, ask your server for uncooked options. The best places will even make special dishes for you that aren't on the menu. If you're willing to inquire, you will find that there is something wonderful waiting for you everywhere you go. The one thing that everyone has in the kitchen—just before they cook it—is living food.

Investigate, ask questions about cleansing and the living foods lifestyle in general. Be your own scientist and health coach, seeking answers for the hows and whys.

At the same time, ask for and be open to receiving support. Seek validation by going to the experts to make sense of your experiences. Be open to answers to why certain thoughts, feelings, and sensations might arise.

In addition to the recipes contained in this book, you can find many more living food recipes at www.brigittemars.com, www.rainbeaumarslifestyles.com, and of course, all over the Internet. There are so many resources on the web just waiting for you—simply ask and you shall receive.

Regardless of how your first day of living foods goes, whether it's smooth sailing or a bumpy ride, see if you can take one step further. Think of it this way: each time we refrain from instant gratification, we receive more light. This adds to our wellspring of positive energy and further strengthens our potential. Wildly successful people know this truth. Nothing really life changing comes without work on our part. I know with certainty that if you hold a vision of the inevitable outcome, it is entirely worth it.

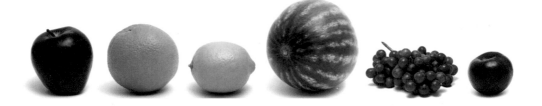

EAT THE RAINBOW

COLORS	FOODS	COLORFUL PROTECTIVE SUBSTANCES & POSSIBLE ACTIONS
Red	tomato and tomato products, watermelon, guava	lycopene: antioxidant; cuts prostate cancer risk
Orange	carrot, yam, sweet potato, mango, pumpkin	beta-carotene: supports immune system; powerful antioxidant
Yellow-Orange	citrus fruits: orange, lemon, grapefruit, papaya, peach	vitamin C, flavonoids: inhibit tumor cell growth; detoxify harmful substances (free radicals)
Green	spinach, kale, collard, and other greens	folate: supports healthy cell growth
Green-White	broccoli, brussels sprouts, cabbage, cauliflower	indoles, lutein: eliminate excess estrogen and carcinogens
White-Green	garlic, onion, chive, asparagus	allyl sulfides: destroy cancer cells, reduce cell division, support immune system
Blue	blueberries, purple grapes, plums	anthocyanins: destroy free radicals
Red-Purple	grapes, berries, plums, dragon fruit	resveratrol: may decrease estrogen production
Brown	whole grains, legumes	fiber: removes carcinogens

BENEFITS OF LIVE FOODS

- Live foods are simple to make, removing the step of cooking and the difficulty of cleaning gooey, burned pots and pans.
- You can dehydrate, marinate, and soak in order to prepare dishes and render them more digestible, without ever having to worry about burning the house down.
- Live food is more than just uncooked—it is a way to define nourishing, whole foods that are brimming with nutrients, including a massive amount of enzymes that support optimal digestion.
- If we are what you eat, then eating live foods will leave you more vibrant, energetic, and well … *alive!!!*
- Live foods are everywhere, in every restaurant all the time. You simply have to intervene before the food is chemically changed, rendered devoid of enzymes, and filled with free-radical-producing oils.
- Live foods from plants, trees, and bushes do not require factories, plastics, chemicals, or a refinement process. Nature provides food that is easy to use, offering nourishment just the way our bodies need.
- Living foods provide enzymes, which reduce inflammation and allow the intestines, liver, and pancreas to better do their jobs.
- Live foods like sprouts, seeds, fruits, and vegetables are high in fiber and water, both hydrating our bodies and sweeping out our intestines so we can better absorb the nutrients we consume.
- The more we align with nature, the more beautiful we are and the more we attract all that is great into our lives—including abundance, prosperity, love, health, and wealth on every level (physically, emotionally, mentally, and spiritually). This is the Law of Attraction in action.

Note: See "Ten More Reasons to Go Raw" in Rainbeau's Reading Room on page 356 for further motivation for the living foods lifestyle.

ENZYMES IN LIVING FOODS

Enzymes are the proteins that increase or decrease every reaction in our body. Every interaction between cells, every thought and every action within our body, involves enzymes. The body's ability to function properly and in an optimal state depends in great part on its stores of enzymes.

In 1878, the German physician, philosopher, and psychology professor Wilhelm Kühne coined the word "enzyme" to specify this increase or decrease in chemical reactions—the biocatalyst actions—that originate outside a living cell. It is interesting to note that the word enzyme actually means "to liven." Understanding how enzymes interact with our body and increase our health gives us the foundation for knowing how to "liven" to our greatest potential. As enzymes are the "living sparks" needed for every chemical action and reaction in the body, it seems only natural to reach the conclusion that by eating foods that are full of enzymes, we are giving our bodies the necessary fuel for harmonious intercellular communication and organ function.

Certain enzymes are produced in the body (endogenous), and some come from outside the body (exogenous). That is to say, digestive enzymes within our bodies are not the same as the enzymes in raw, unprocessed food. Digestive enzymes break down the complex substances we ingest into simple components the body can utilize. There are five types of digestive enzymes in the human body:

- *Hydrolases* facilitate hydrolysis, the breakdown of substances in water.
- *Adding enzymes* build proteins by adding amino acids.
- *Transferring enzymes* transfer organic substances from one compound to another so the body can use them in various ways.
- *Isomerases*, or *rearranging enzymes*, rearrange molecules and amino acids.
- *Oxidases*, or *oxidizing enzymes*, are released in the presence of oxygen. They act on foods in the mouth while one is masticating (chewing) or whenever the food is exposed to oxygen. These enzymes are also present in apples and other fruits and are released when the fruit is cut, rapidly bringing about a change of color—the browning of an apple, for example.

Outside of the human body, enzymes are present everywhere, sprouting up from the rich earth and falling from the branches of generous trees and bushes. With its own enzymes, an apple immediately starts to break itself down without any help from the body's store of enzymes. Imagine how much easier it is on the body to consume this live food as opposed to a cooked apple that no longer has any enzyme activity. Our body must work twice as hard to create the complementary enzymes to break it down.

When we eat living foods, we feel energized because the body doesn't have to work as hard to digest our food. Enzymes work together to bring us the nutrients we need to thrive. In that sense, enzymes are one of the keys to experiencing the benefts this SuperStar Cleanse.

ENZYMES IN ACTION

ORGAN	SUBSTANCE	ACTS ON	FINAL PRODUCT
Mouth	· Salivary amalyse	· Starch	· Maltose *(disaccharides)*
Stomach	· Pepsin · Hydrochloric acid *(produced by lining)*	· Protein · Acidity needed for pepsin and to kill bacteria	· Polypeptides · Creates digestive medium
Duodenum *(first part of the small intestine)*	· Secretin · Pancreozymin	· Stimulates flow of pancreatic juices · Stimulates production of enzymes	· Receives enzymes from pancreas and liver
Pancreas	· Amylase · Lipase · Protease *(trypsin)*	· Starch, glycogen · Protein · Emulsified fats	· Maltose · Fatty acids, glycerol · Amino acids—polypeptides, peptides
Small Intestine *(secreted by glands in lining)*	· Maltase · Sucrase · Lactase	· Disaccharides · Sucrose · Lactose	· Monosaccharides · Glucose · Fructose
Liver & Gallbladder	· Bile salts	· Large fat globules	· Emulsified fats—fatty acids
Large Intestine	· Bacteria	· Undigested food · Water and salt	· Water · Dead cells

MORE REASONS TO EAT ENZYMES

Minerals, vitamins, and hormones cannot be distributed throughout the body or absorbed into the body except in the presence of enzymes. This means that when you have enzymes in your body, you are absorbing the necessary minerals and vitamins for vibrant health.

Enzymes assist in the regulation of hormones and help synthesize and duplicate entire chains of amino acids—the building blocks of protein.

Enzymes have been used with great success in treatment of arthritis, auto-immune disorders, cancers, viral infections, varicose veins, fat intolerance, cystic fibrosis, autism, sports injuries, and pain reduction.

Decreased enzyme activity has been found to contribute to chronic conditions such as allergies, skin disease, diabetes, and cancer.

Lack of enzymes can also contribute to weight gain, lethargy, depression, digestive impairment, and loss of skin elasticity and muscle tone, which are symptoms of aging.

When enzyme function is impaired, our body has to work harder to accomplish normal metabolic processes, and we begin to age prematurely and unnecessarily. Getting older does not mean our health has to fail.

Plant a raw sunflower seed, and it will grow into a ten-foot-tall plant with a bright beaming flower that results in hundreds of seeds. Plant a roasted sunflower seed and it rots in the ground. The difference? Enzymes!

In short, breathing, sleeping, eating, digestion, nutrient absorption, thinking, moving, working, immune function, reproduction, sexual activity, dreaming, sensory perception, and more *are all dependent on enzymes*. Each interaction that requires communication between cells relies on the presence of enzymes in the body.

THE LIVE FOODS KITCHEN

Activation

The kitchen is the center of the home. When I support friends and clients in person, one of the first things we do together is "activate" the kitchen. Preparing them for their new lifestyle involves opening up the drawers and cupboards that also serve as potent metaphors. The kitchen is a reliable mirror of key elements of our lives. In a very tangible way, it functions as the core of our experience of self and how we relate to our community and the planet. To activate your own kitchen, consider clearing out packaged, old, or toxic foods, chipped plates and glasses, peeling Teflon pans, and clutter you no longer need. Also, doing a deeper level of cleaning and bringing in some fresh flowers or a plant are easy ways to infuse your kitchen with more beauty and love.

Hearth and Home

An icon of the kitchen is the flame, that elemental force that throughout history has been both the savior and demise of the tribe. For use in cooking, work, warmth, and protection, fire has been imperative to our survival. But like all forces of nature, when it is out of our control, that same life-giving fire can become destructive and wipe out necessary resources. In the live foods kitchen, one of the ways we cultivate balance with the Fire element is through the practice of not heating foods above 118° F in order to protect their vital nutrients and enzymes.

Naturally Perfect

Another restorative aspect of the live food diet is that it puts us in communion with the inherent forces of nature. In the live food kitchen, we are constantly sprouting, growing, and touching the soil that is like nature's womb, holding the seedlings that will blossom into their fullness. We realign with nature's rhythms when we eat foods that are grown locally and when we prepare and cook with ingredients that are in season. Growing a garden is an excellent idea. Herb gardens can be grown in even the most urban settings with the right garden box, earth, water, and sunshine. Not only will you then have access to the freshest herbs possible, you'll also have ingredients that resonate with your unique energy. The more we commune with the grace of Mother Earth, the less stress we experience. We too are capable of emanating nature's exquisite qualities of perfection.

Transitioning

Fresh foods are always best, but when we feel the need for foods that have the density or warmth of cooked foods, there are simple and accessible solutions. Dehydration is a helpful method of "unplugging" from cooking your food. One simple example is using a dehydrator to make raw crackers that are packed with nutrition, calories, and crunch. On the stove top, cooked wild rice, quinoa, and squash are good winter transition foods as they retain many nutrients even when lightly cooked. Try soaking your grains over night and then rinsing them, resulting in far less cooking.

As you progress on your journey into the world of living foods, notice which foods work for you and which you'd do better to avoid. Just because it's raw doesn't mean it will be nourishing or easy to digest. For example, try to avoid starches (which contain double-bonded sugars) such as potatoes, grains, noodles, and other hybridized foods like corn and beans that are difficult for the body to recognize and digest.

A special note about frozen foods and doing your best: Although many of us delight in the creamy sensation of cold smoothies and ice creams, it's important to remember that we lose half the enzymes when we freeze our food. So consider using your foods fresh and garnishing with cooler or cold toppings for fun. For example, you could have a bowl of fresh peaches garnished with coconut or cashew whipped cream.

REFLECTIONS
discovering yourself anew

In your journal or on your computer, continue your process of introspection and reflection through writing. Think about the questions below, meditate, and write. Take this time for self-inquiry as you shift and transform.

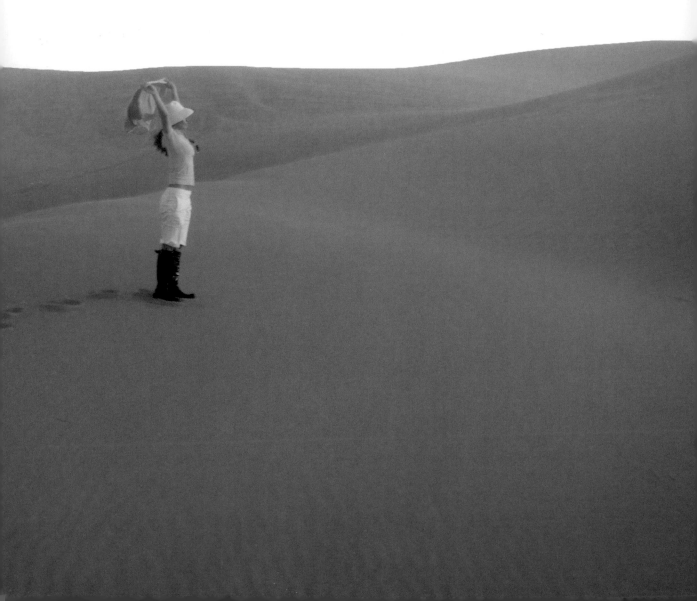

1. How has adding live foods to your diet impacted your body or mind this week? How has it made you feel? Any new sensations? With all of the additional enzymes, did you notice any changes in your digestion?

2. Were there any particular cravings that arose? Were these cravings for certain foods, feelings, relationships, places, or activities?

3. What moods and emotions did you experience? Were you able to be present with those emotions?

4. Were you aware of any limiting thoughts or beliefs this week?

5. How easy or challenging was it to follow through with this week's recommendations and guidelines?

6. Which recipes, action steps, or tips did you incorporate? And how did it feel to increase your self-care?

7. How did your body feel when you exercised? Did you notice areas where you were more flexible? Have any areas of tension decreased?

8. Have your sleep patterns changed? Did you sleep less or more?

9. If by chance you were not able to exactly stick to the program (or even thought about cheating), were you okay with that, or did you let judgments and feelings of failure arise to the point of strengthening the negativity? We will all fall asleep, but we become stronger when we wake up more quickly.

10. Do you find yourself aspiring for something higher in your thoughts, visions, and actions? Are you focusing on and remembering your intentions at all times?

WHAT THE EYES
ARE FOR THE
OUTER WORLD,
FASTS ARE FOR
THE INNER.

—GANDHI

CHAPTER 4

WEEK THREE: THE BLENDED FOODS BREAKTHROUGH

A few years ago, I decided to incorporate an adapted version of the twenty-one-day cleanse program to a yoga teacher training I was leading. Wonderful women and men were coming in from all over the world, and I wanted to share with them the program that I had received so many benefits from. They each expressed enthusiasm for doing the cleanse and for eating vegan and live, blended foods during the training—so we went for it. We were off and running, and what a memorable time we would end up having together! In some ways, being away from their normal routines made it easier for people to dive into the experience. And, as you might imagine, that same break from normal routine and surroundings had some people craving the familiar—like the familiar fried *this* or animal products *that*. And the familiar glass of wine and cup of coffee. I could safely say that just about all of us were invited to embrace the edge, to step into and through some uncomfortable territory (physically, mentally, and emotionally) on the way to the greater levels of aliveness that awaited us. There were a few times when I seriously questioned whether we had done the right thing in merging the training with the cleanse

(I'll share another story later in the book that illustrates one of those moments!), but it turned out that our instincts were trustworthy. The vibrance and vitality of the organic live foods, coupled with the practice of yoga, was profoundly uplifting and replenishing ... positively altering lives in the particular way that was meaningful to each person. In the end, the rapid increase in energy and health that took place for all of us, due in large part to the rejuvenating power of blended foods, helped us let go of the old and prepare for the new and unknown. This is something I have watched happen with hundreds of others as well. Blended foods are an amazing addition to the plan or blueprint of a lifetime of radiance that I described in the beginning of this book.

So, are you ready to pick up the pace of healing change?

By consuming blended foods all week—or as much as possible, depending on how you're choosing to customize your program—the goal is to ease the constant burden you tend to place on your digestive system. You won't be sacrificing calories or giving up anything (other than chewing). The beauty of blended food is that it has already been "pre-digested," meaning that the blending process breaks down the cell walls in food, making all the nutrients readily available to the body and extremely easy to digest so more nutrients can be absorbed. As a result, the body has more metabolic and digestive energy available for other functions. I have also found that everyone especially loves this week because of the truly mind-blowing inner and outer transformation that takes place, as it typically results in a flat, beach-ready tummy!

Also, imagine the extra time you will have—time for beauty disciplines, to complete tasks, finish that script or book, plant those seeds, meditate, or include more exercise in your day. This is the time you would have used to cook, clean, and recover from the effects of cooked foods.

Last week, you received a preview of this week's many blended options. This week you will have the opportunity to continue that exploration, which includes amazing live soups, blended desserts and puddings, veggie and fruit purees, shakes, smoothies, guacamole and other dips, and nut and seed chees-es. You can incorporate as many blended foods as you like each day, whether you choose to have one blended meal per day or the majority of them blended. Basically, the more blended meals you include this week, the faster you will see results. And regardless of how you choose to tailor your program, even if you decide that you need to include some of the lightly cooked vegan meals from Week One, the most important thing is to incorporate as much fresh, liv-ing produce into your menu as you can (remembering that eating cooked food does stop the cleansing process).

Now, this is also the week where you may opt to fast for one day or more. The choice is yours. Remember: if this is your first round with *The 21-Day SuperStar Cleanse*, you may decide to eat all blended foods the next round. Challenge yourself to be healthier, yet love yourself *through* the process. This is not meant to be restrictive or torturous! Quite the contrary: this is a gentle stripping down of layers no longer needed on your way to internal and external health and beauty. When you abstain from addictive and detrimental foods, certain crav-ings are likely to make themselves known. So, allow yourself to observe what arises, and breathe through the "I must have that now!" moments. These are the moments that seduce us into giving in to temptation and, sadly, block us from our goals. Each day, quietly reflect and intuitively choose what feels per-fect for *you, your body,* and *your process* at this point in time. Do your best to focus on your intention to finish the program and reap all the rewards.

It is worth saying again and again: healing, health, and happiness come from the inside out. Consider the Law of Attraction for a moment: if what you de-sire in your life is beauty, truth, health, and abundance, you must surround yourself inside and out with beauty, truth, health, and abundance. This is how you can directly shift your internal world to attract what you desire on the outside. And your commitment to your twenty-one-day program will make it so. And so it is ... let's begin Week Three!

CHANNELS OF ENERGY AND LIGHT
week three

The Way of Light

During the first two weeks of the program, you brought your awareness to the subtle channels of energy (the *nadis*) known as the *ida* and *pingala*, the feminine and masculine principles, the yin and yang that we animate externally and internally. This week, in sync with the radiant energy that is unleashed when you take in more living blended foods and juices, you are primed to call on the energy of *sushumna,* the balance of the feminine and masculine principles that corresponds with the center of the body. Associated in the outer world with the ancient river Saraswati, internally the *sushumna* represents the way of light that becomes more accessible when you consciously engage in an extended cleansing program such as this. In Kundalini Yoga, balancing *ida* and *pingala* invites *prana* (vital life force enegy) to flow through the channel of *sushumna* and is essential preparation for Kundalini awakening. This is the energetic pathway of physical and spiritual enlightenment—where two become one.

Toward the full awakening of your body and mind this week, observe the balance of energy within you. Notice how fasting with living foods moves your energy upward and supports your internal alignment. Remember: the energy and direction we want to travel is up.

CUSTOMIZING YOUR SUPERSTAR PLAN
week three

Whether you're new to blended foods or a seasoned lover of them, I assure you that you won't be bored! In addition to the pleasures of life-giving water, herbal teas, and fresh, organic juices, you can enjoy blended soups, smoothies, shakes, dips, cheeses, guacs, and even chocolate mousse and other blended desserts that are *ridiculously* delicious. It brings me great satisfaction to indulge in lemon meringue pie and tiramisu for my beauty and blended diet.

FOR THE BEGINNER
Depending on what feels right for you, you might choose to make this another week of all live foods, or maybe this is your *first* week of living foods. Perhaps you decided to have the past week be another seven days of lightly cooked vegan dishes. Start from wherever you are and be willing to take another step forward. Blend for at least one or two days, if you can.

FOR THE INTERMEDIATE
Eat, drink, and chew almost all blended foods, with one to two days that incorporate raw, living foods that are not strictly blended. Basically, consume as much blended food as possible, but be happy to "cheat" with pieces of fruit or other live snacks in between.

FOR THE ADVANCED
I invite you to stick to *all* blended live foods. Also consider selecting one or two days to be traditional fasting days, where you drink only water, teas, and juices or potentially a gallbladder cleanse.

FOR EVERYONE
From beginner to advanced, enjoy the adventure that awaits you on the inside of your blessed blender. From the humblest to the most powerful, our blenders can whip up some unbelievably nutritious magic.

PREPARING FOR YOUR SUPERSTAR CLEANSE
week three

The week that you are stepping into can be one of the most transforming and enlightening weeks of your life so far. I encourage you to use the daily and weekly guidelines and suggestions to get the most you can out of each day. Open your body and mind to the possibility that continuing your cleanse with gusto can lead to a new sense of enchantment in your life. Energy and health have a way of putting a shimmer around just about *everything*.

STEP 1

If applicable, please read and consider supplementing your program with the following sections found in Rainbeau's Reading Room:

1. 28 Beauty Rituals on page 370.
2. Introduction to Colon Hydrotherapy and Enema Instructions on pages 377 and 380. Enemas are encouraged up to twice a day in some cases, so make time for them ... and let go of the past. The yogis who live in healthy physical freedom at old ages are testaments to these practices.

STEP 2

Each morning, begin by reviewing the Toolkit for that day. Commit to incorporating at least one suggestion. Choose those that make you *feel* something inside.

STEP 3

Journal about blended foods experiences this week, and contemplate how you can incorporate more blended foods into your lifestyle after you've completed the twenty-one-day program.

STEP 4

Are you ready to try a radical beauty technique? It's one of my favorites. I invite you to designate at least one day this week as a Self-Care Day. You've been fitting in self-care minutes and hours, so now is a good time to further expand that quality *you* time. It doesn't need to be *all* day, but choose at least two activities that you schedule into the same day. Consider a "beauty-and-care me day," where the schedule consists of a facial, a colonic, a restorative yoga class, a long, lingering candle lit bath, or any other items from the 28 Beauty Rituals section in Rainbeau's Reading Room.

In addition, for this entire day, *speak and think only positive words of love to yourself*. If you do have a negative thought, course-correct by saying at least three positive affirmations about yourself for every negative thought that arises.

Whatever we focus on expands. What kind of focus do you bring to yourself today? Do you love your eyes, lips, legs, hair, smile, skin, stomach, kindness, empathy, or patience? Focus on all that you *love*, and let that spread to the rest of you, which will allow you to pass that irresistible glow on to others as well. Every time you see yourself in a mirror on this special day, blow yourself a kiss and declare, *I love you!* (I can see you smiling already.)

SPEAK ONLY POSITIVE WORDS OF LOVE TO YOURSELF.

SHOPPING LIST
and general food guidelines

Going back to the benefits of fasting, this is the part of the program where we break patterns of addiction, a time when we get in touch with who we really are, along with our sensitivities and our abilities to *heal ourselves*. These are the guidelines for a successful blended food extravaganza. I encourage you with all my heart to proceed lightly, with a commitment to yourself to remember that *nothing tastes as good as feeling good feels.*

In addition to some of the items you have already purchased, you'll want to have a ready supply of the following ripe living foods on hand, and you will want to remain well stocked.

HERBS, FRUITS, & VEGGIES
- Avocados (7 to 14)
- Bananas
- Basil
- Beets
- Bell peppers
- Blackberries
- Blueberries
- Carrots
- Celery
- Cilantro
- Coconuts (one case of young Thai coconuts)
- Dates
- Dill
- Garlic
- Ginger, fresh
- Greens, including dark, leafy greens such as collards, kale, spinach, or other
- Lavender (for tea)
- Lemons
- Mangos
- Mint
- Oranges
- Parsley
- Red raspberry leaf (for tea)
- Rosemary
- Strawberries
- Sprouts (sunflower, broccoli, or other)
- Seaweeds, (arame, dulse, and Irish moss)
- Tomatoes
- Watermelon

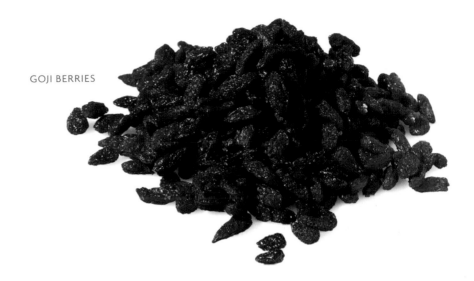

GOJI BERRIES

NUTS

- Almonds
- Brazil nuts
- Cashews
- Macadamias

SPICES

- Cayenne
- Cumin
- Cinnamon
- Chili powder
- Curry
- Vanilla

CONDIMENTS

- Bragg Liquid Aminos
- Celtic sea salt
- Miso, unpasteurized
- Olive oil, organic extra-virgin, stored in a dark glass bottle and away from heat

SPECIALTY FOODS

- Barley grass powder
- Cacao powder, raw
- Chia seeds
- Goji berry powder
- Maca
- Superfood supplement for use in everything: HealthForce Vitamineral Green or HealthForce Vitamineral Earth
- Shaman Shack Herbs: Sea Clear, 3 Immortals, and 3 Jewels

BEST PRACTICES
for week three

WATERMELON DAY

If it's in season, choose one day to fast with watermelon and lemon water, with an extra kick of cayenne and some sweetener to enhance circulation. The best watermelons have seeds, which are an incredible kidney tonic—so chew them up and swallow.

FRUIT-ONLY MEALS

Combine any of your favorite fruits—in the quantities you want—to make delicious meal substitutes that are high in nutrients and natural sugars to keep you energized.

Examples:

- 1 bunch of bananas
- 3 mangos
- Big basket of strawberries
- Bag of oranges
- 1 container of dates
- A bowl of blueberries or blackberries

CHOCOLATE BLISS

You may choose chocolate smoothies every other day. However, since we can overdo anything, even healthy things, remember that *conscious* indulgence is an important part of this healing journey.

JUICE FASTING

You have the option of juicing for one or two days. Make or order juices that are high in celery, greens, and cooling cucumber. If you take this option, you are also welcome to add some olive oil and even a little Himalayan pink salt or Celtic sea salt to your juices.

ENERGY SOUP

Energy Soup may be just the solution! The following is simply a base line and it's suggested that you try everything. Miso, lemon and sprouts seem to always help!

INGREDIENTS

- 1 avocado
- 1 carrot
- 1 to 2 tomatoes
- 1 lemon
- 1 bunch of sprouts
- 1 bunch of kale
- Peppers of your choice
- Sliver of papaya
- Cilantro, basil, or any other preferred fresh herbs
- Himalayan or Celtic salt
- Unpasteurized miso
- 1 handful of soaked raw almonds
- 1 small handful of your favorite seaweed

DIRECTIONS

1. In your blender, mix your choice of ingredients at a pulse, taking care not to overblend.
2. Create any version of this you like for real, live energy!

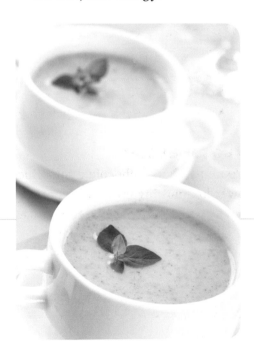

DAY FIFTEEN **SCHEDULE**

7:00 AM	DAWN GLOW TONIC Liver Kick (page 94) Nettles tea
8:00 AM	BREAKFAST Coconut Delight (page 333)
10:00 AM	YOGA POSE OF THE DAY Option: *ra'yoKa* Sequence of the Day Option: Take a brisk walk with a friend or by yourself
12:00 NOON	LUNCH Recipe of the Day: Butterscotch Pudding (page 326) Option: Live Chocolate Shake (page 334)
1:00 PM	SELF-TLC Option: Create a Week Three vision board (collage) of your goals, or add to one you've already started Option: Contemplate today's action step for Aligning with Your Ultimate Purpose

DAY 15 ★

4:00 PM	**DINNER** Energy Soup (page 315) Option: Guacamole (page 321)
6:00 PM	**GET YOUR GLOW ON** Put your legs up the wall and listen to music or read for fifteen minutes
AS DESIRED	**SNACKS & DESSERTS** Drink more juice—consider fasting for the whole day. Warm Maca Mocha 'n' Cinnamon (page 337) (*Note: Try to keep chocolate goodies down to one per day*)
7:00 PM	**DUSK GLOW TONIC** Enjoy fresh lavender and chamomile tea to calm the system Consider drinking this while soaking in a bath with the same herbs

SUPPLEMENTAL RECOMMENDATION

Chew holy basil for a feeling of openness and euphoria—and you get to chew!

DAY FIFTEEN **TOOLKIT**

Virtue of the Day: *Altruism*

As you increase your energy this week with blended foods and juices and healing tonics, you are likely to discover a natural desire to reach out to others in service and support. Today, allow your attention to dwell upon the energy of altruism, a devotion to the welfare of others. Altruism is your social conscience generously put into action. As you blend your recipes and go through your day, allow yourself to give expression to the affectionate selflessness that is alive and well within you.

Action Step of the Day: *Aligning with Your Ultimate Purpose*

An important intention this week is to remain grounded, solidly centered in yourself as you're lightening your body and mind with living foods. As you embark on the final cleansing phase of *The 21-Day SuperStar Cleanse* program, the commitment to blended foods can seem daunting, but remember: you are not in this alone. In addition to our online support community and your personal circle of loved ones, nature herself is encouraging your mission of alignment, evolution, and healing.

We are intrinsically connected to the earth, including its cycles and energies. Whether we refer to it as *prana, chi, ki*, spirit, or life force, we are electrical beings, and this energy—which flows from the earth through us—is an incredibly powerful resource for good health. In the book *Earthing*, Dr. Stephen Sinatra brilliantly illuminates this phenomenon, explains that people in industrialized societies are not fully connecting with the earth's natural electrical currents, and suggests what we can do about it. In essence, we are collectively suffering the adverse effects of being out of sync with the cycles of nature. For example, the sole of the foot has more nerve endings inch for

RECIPE OF THE DAY: **BUTTERSCOTCH PUDDING**

Indulgence, purity, and beauty coexist in this blended treat. Delight in it for breakfast or dessert.

INGREDIENTS

- 1 cup dried apricots, soaked overnight in water (reserve soaking water for blending)
- 2 ripe peeled bananas
- 8 dates, pitted and soaked
- 1 teaspoon vanilla extract
- ¼ cup raw almond butter
- Hint of butterscotch extract, if available (optional)

DIRECTIONS

Process in the food processor with an "S" blade. (4 servings)

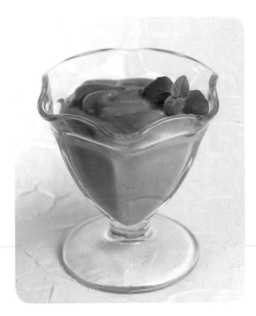

DAY FIFTEEN **TOOLKIT**

inch than any other part of the body, yet when we walk around in rubber-soled shoes or live and work in high-rise buildings, these nerves are unable to connect with the earth. Many indigenous cultures recognize the healing and balancing the earth provides and stay consciously connected by walking barefoot and sleeping on or near the ground.

On the other hand, the energy spectrum in our modern society also includes "dirty electricity," which is formed by an overabundance of electromagnetic fields (or EMFs) present in the atmosphere due to our high-density technology—our ubiquitous cell phones, computers, and WiFi.

Hungry for the natural currents of healing and oversaturated with the human-made currents, our sense of having a solid, secure foundation and flowing life force energy may be impaired—but there are many things we can do to correct the imbalance.

EASY WAYS TO STAY GROUNDED

- Lean against a tree for twenty to thirty minutes. As we rest with the tree, we absorb its grounding energy from the earth. Don't be afraid to hug the tree as well, for further balancing.

- Walk barefoot in nature. Damp grass feels great against the feet and helps conduct electromagnetic energy through the body.

- Being barefoot in salt water (the ocean or a warm salt bath) is highly conductive, elegantly circulating the earth's balancing currents.

- Consider using a mat for your computer or grounding sheets for your bed. I love the BioMat and have been looking into microcirculation mats or magnetic options.

- As I suggested earlier, consider sleeping on a bed that is closer to the ground with, of course, nothing underneath (clear the "parking lot" of things like stacks of paper, books, clothes, or shoes).

Be mindful of the electricity in your home:

- Be sure to check that the electrical outlets in your home are grounded.

- Switch from a cordless phone modem to a landline (to reduce the WiFi electro-pollution).

- Limit cell phone use. When it is necessary to do so, use a special cord or the speakerphone option.

- Avoid wearing the cell phone on your body and turn it off whenever possible.

- Clear the space near your bed of any electronics before you go to sleep at night. (Try a retro wind-up alarm clock.)

- Throughout your home, and especially in your bedroom, plug electronics into smart strips and turn them off at night.

DAY FIFTEEN **TOOLKIT**

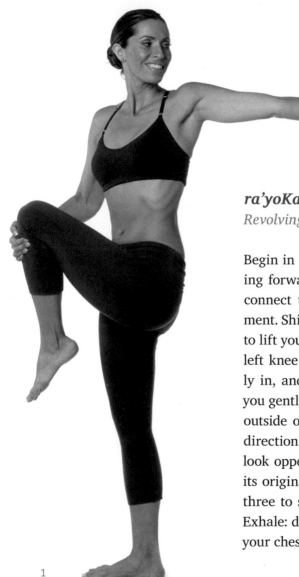

1

ra'yoKa Sequence of the Day:
Revolving Knee to Chest

Begin in *Tadasana*—heels in a line, big toes facing forward. Spread your toes, firm your body, connect to your core, and maintain the alignment. Shift your weight to your right foot. Inhale to lift your chest, and on your exhale bring your left knee in toward your chest. Draw your belly in, and avoid overstretching the neck while you gently revolve the knee outward toward the outside of your body and look in the opposite direction. Exhale, twist the knee outward, and look opposite. Inhale, bring the knee back into its original position, and repeat this movement three to six times. The breath is fluid and full. Exhale: draw in your belly and twist. Inhale: lift your chest and return to your original position.

226

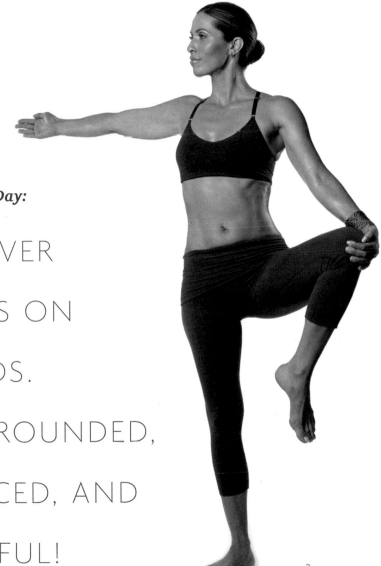

Mantra of the Day:

WHATEVER I FOCUS ON EXPANDS. I AM GROUNDED, BALANCED, AND BEAUTIFUL!

2

DAY SIXTEEN SCHEDULE

7:00 AM   DAWN GLOW TONIC
Start with liver tonic of your choice
Caffeine-free chai with raw almond milk

8:00 AM   BREAKFAST
Recipe of the Day: Banana Almond Shake with Ginger
(page 331)
Option: Chia Pudding (page 326) with raw almond milk,
sprinkled with flaxseeds and cinnamon

10:00 AM   YOGA POSE OF THE DAY
Option: *Yoga for Beauty* Pose of the Day
Option: Twenty-minute meditation or a walk in nature

12:00 NOON   LUNCH
Energy Soup (page 315)

1:00 PM   SELF-TLC
Option: Read an inspiring passage from a book
Option: Contemplate today's action step for Aligning with
Your Ultimate Purpose

DAY **16** ★

4:00 PM	DINNER
	Raw Cooling Gazpacho (page 317)

6:00 PM	YOGA POSE OF THE DAY
	Treat yourself to a luxurious Beauty Bath. See the Superstar Skin section on page 274 to find your head-to toe glow.

AS DESIRED	SNACKS & DESSERTS
	1 cup of Live Chocolate Pudding (page 327)

7:00 PM	DUSK GLOW TONIC
	Tea of nettles and red raspberry to support the kidneys and hormones

SUPPLEMENTAL RECOMMENDATION

Consider enhancing your cleanse with a little extra chlorophyll. It may not be a totally raw food, but it does alkalize the system and makes you feel so good and fresh that you'll stick to the plan. In addition to the chlorophyll in your leafy green vegetables and green juices, you can also buy a bottle of chlorophyll and add some to your water.

Also, consider using chlorophyll in enemas (hopefully, you're doing them daily). You could alternate between enemas that include organic deacidified coffee and good water in the morning and/or chlorophyll in the evening.

DAY SIXTEEN TOOLKIT

Virtue of the Day: *Philanthropy*

Energetically, today aligns with yesterday as an opportunity to place some of your attention on other people's welfare and advancement. Although philanthropy is often associated with financial giving to organizations and individuals, at the heart of it, philanthropy is the act of donating anything that brings relief to and uplifts others. As you sip on a juice or herbal tea today, see if there is one thing you could donate, whether that gift is financial, material, intellectual, emotional, or creative in nature.

Action Step of the Day: *Aligning with Your Ultimate Purpose*

In keeping with the theme of grounding and "earthing" this week, this is a good day to learn about easy composting. We are all stewards of this communal garden we call Earth, and as we practice what I like to call mindful habits, we can conserve our precious natural resources while promoting future abundance. Imagine if all you ever did with your bank account was withdraw from it? Consider Earth's minerals in the same way. We must give back in order for it to keep giving to us.

Attuning us to nature's rhythms in very practical ways, composting is a mindful habit that is both environmentally and economically beneficial. It cleans up contaminated soil, reduces waste, curbs greenhouse gases, helps prevent pollution and erosion, saves money, and supports the growth of lush organic gardens through enrichment of our soil.

This week your live and blended foods lifestyle will likely produce a lot of food scraps for composting. But not to worry—you don't need a big yard to start churning out your own compost. Even the most restricted urban homesteaders

DAY 16

RECIPE OF THE DAY: BANANA ALMOND SHAKE WITH GINGER

This creamy goodness is simply Nirvana in a glass.

INGREDIENTS

- 1 cup almond milk
- 1 ripe banana
- 2 soaked dates
- 1 teaspoon vanilla extract (optional)
- 2 tablespoons almond butter (optional)
- 1 inch of fresh ginger

DIRECTIONS

Blend all ingredients and enjoy. (1 serving)

INGREDIENTS—ALMOND MILK

- 1 cup almonds, soaked overnight and rinsed
- 1 quart of pure water
- 1 teaspoon raw honey or 2 dates, soaked

DIRECTIONS—ALMOND MILK

1. Blend almond milk ingredients.
2. Strain through a nut milk bag, sprout bag, or strainer.
   Makes 1 quart.

Note: When making nut milk, save the pulp for making cheese. These same directions can be used for making cashew, hazelnut, sesame, sunflower, walnut, or pecan milk.

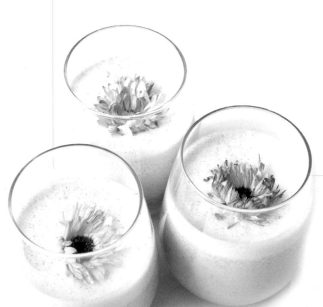

DAY SIXTEEN TOOLKIT

can partake of this sustainable practice, utilizing space-conservative methods like the following:

FERMENTATION

The Bokashi-style system uses microbes and wheat bran to anaerobically ferment organic waste. You can add the scraps to a worm bin or bury them directly in the soil. Perfect for apartments or offices, these closed-system containers keep out undesirable insects and keep in smells.

VERMICOMPOSTING

This method uses the digestive talents of earthworms to break down organic matter into dark, earthy compost that is brimming with planet-loving nutrients. It can be easily made from an eight- to ten-gallon opaque storage container.

MECHANIZED COMPOSTER

The size of a regular trashcan, it can be stowed away in any standard cabinet if you're short on square footage. The electric composter mixes, heats, and aerates food scraps, then transfers the contents into a lower chamber that produces fresh, garden-ready compost after two weeks.

WAYS TO USE YOUR FINISHED COMPOST

- Add a bit to the surface of your houseplant pots or combine with potting soil or seed-starting mixes.
- Donate your compost to a community garden, school garden, or garden club.
- Guerilla gardening soil improvement: add your compost to public plantings where appropriate to help them grow stronger.
- Make an offer—sell compost online.

Yoga for Beauty Pose of the Day: *Extended Right Angle*

Begin in Warrior Two with your left leg forward. Your front left heel should be in line with the arch of your back right foot. Back foot is at a ninety-degree angle. Reach forward with your front left hand, hinge from the hips. Bring the left elbow to your knee and inhale, reaching the right arm over into a side stretch. Reverse out the way you came in and make sure you switch sides with your right leg forward. Take at least five breaths on each side.

Mantra of the Day: TODAY IS A SACRED GIFT FROM LIFE.

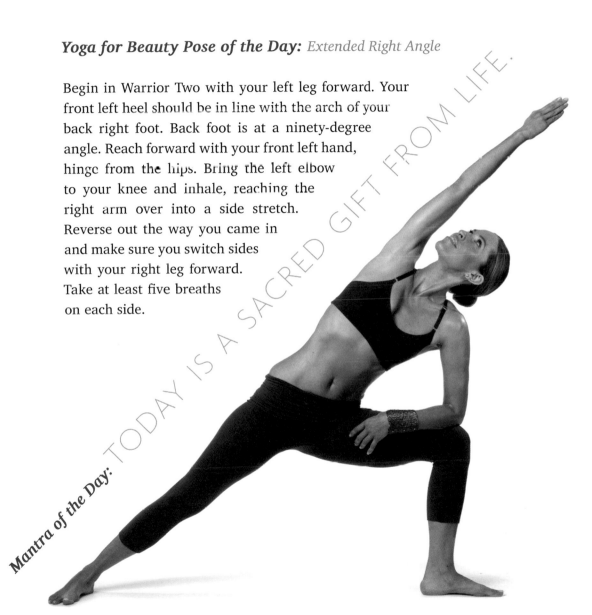

DAY SEVENTEEN SCHEDULE

7:00 AM DAWN GLOW TONIC
Start with liver tonic of your choice

8:00 AM BREAKFAST
Recipe of the Day: Raw Kiwi-Lime Coconut Pie (page 329)
Option: 1 Live Chocolate Shake (page 334) with almond milk, raw honey, maca, and Brazil nut powder

10:00 AM YOGA POSE OF THE DAY
Option: *Yoga for Beauty* Pose of the Day
Option: Practice conscious breathing (*pranayama*)

12:00 NOON LUNCH
Easy tomato soup: combine 2 large tomatoes, 1 red bell pepper, 1 date, pinch Celtic sea salt, olive oil, nama shoyu, 1 cup of water, and blend. Spice accordingly

1:00 PM SELF-TLC
Option: Call someone you adore on the phone
Option: Contemplate today's action step for Aligning with Your Ultimate Purpose

4:00 PM	DINNER
	Mexicali Soup (page 316)

6:00 PM	GET YOUR GLOW ON
	Option: Roll around or do summersaults on the grass!
	Option: Take a long bath with candles

AS DESIRED	SNACKS & DESSERTS
	1 cup of hot water with a touch of raw miso paste. Enjoy!

7:00 PM	DUSK GLOW TONIC
	Lemonade (page 334)
	Option: holy basil tea for relaxed rejuvenation

SUPPLEMENTAL RECOMMENDATION

Support and reculture your inner terrain with daily acidophilus, the friendly bacteria discussed earlier (Days Three and Four). This will create an army of internal good guys after you flush out the bad with purifying enemas. Strengthens the immune system and improves the quality and functioning of your inner environment.

DAY SEVENTEEN **TOOLKIT**

Virtue of the Day: *Compassion*

On your third day of Week Three, you may be feeling a new kind of openness to the world. I will join you in this place with a story. Once the Buddha was asked by his attendant, Ananda, "Would it be true to say that cultivation of loving-kindness and compassion is a part of our practice?" To this the Buddha replied, "No. It would not be true to say that the cultivation of loving-kindness and compassion is part of our practice. It would be true to say that the cultivation of loving-kindness and compassion is *all* of our practice." Breathe into that and be on your way ...

Action Step of the Day: *Aligning with Your Ultimate Purpose*

Smile. Nothing says "health" better than a vibrant smile. Just as our eyes are often referred to as the mirrors of our souls, our mouths are often windows into our body's health. Infections, nutritional deficiencies, and some diseases such as diabetes, heart disease, and stroke are often correlated with issues occurring in our mouths. In addition, a misaligned bite affects chewing and digestion, and temporomandibular joint (TMJ) dysfunction can indicate other musculoskeletal problems. Gum disease infects and destroys tissues, ligaments, and bones; it can also dramatically reduce the effectiveness of the immune system and actually shorten life expectancy. It is important to take the time to see the dentist (holistic if possible) and invest in good dental work as necessary. The following are some tips to keep your smile radiant. And as I share them with you, I share them with myself too; I promise to hop on the oral hygiene bandwagon that I have often not made time for. The time is now.

RECIPE OF THE DAY: **RAW KIWI-LIME COCONUT PIE**

This blended bliss combines the brightness of lime and kiwi with the satisfying creaminess of coconut and soaked nuts.

INGREDIENTS—CRUST

- 1 cup walnuts (soaked and rinsed)
- 1 cup macadamia nuts (soaked and rinsed) or all macs and no walnuts.
- ¼ teaspoon Celtic sea salt
- 6 dates
- ¼ teaspoon vanilla (optional)

INGREDIENTS—FILLING

- 2 tablespoons Irish moss (soaked 12 to 24 hours and rinsed)
- 1 fresh kiwi lime (skinned)
- 1½ cup coconut water (young Thai coconut)
- ½ cup coconut meat (young Thai coconut)
- 1 ripe avocado
- ½ cup cashews or macadamia nuts (soaked and rinsed)

- ¼ cup raw honey, maple syrup, or agave nectar (to taste)
- 1 tablespoon fresh lime juice
- 1 teaspoon vanilla
- ⅛ teaspoon Celtic sea salt
- ½ cup coconut butter or coconut oil

DIRECTIONS

1. Combine crust ingredients in a food processor with the "S" blade and mix thoroughly. Remove and press into pie pan.
2. Chill or dehydrate for 5 hours.
3. Add Irish moss and coconut water and blend until smooth.
4. Gradually add remaining filling ingredients, blending until thick and creamy.
5. Pour into pan over prepared piecrust and chill in fridge.
6. When set, garnish with lime slices and serve. Skin and slice the kiwi to display internal ringed pattern in each slice.

DAY SEVENTEEN TOOLKIT

THE MOUTH

The mouth is the opening to the throat. It is an important area that mirrors much of how we present ourselves to the world. For optimal oral health, we can floss, brush regularly, and eat mouth-freshening herbs and gum-strengthening foods. Celery, apples, carrots, parsley, mint tea, and chlorophyll are great breath fresheners. Healthy Gum Drops by Living Libations is a great remedy, potent with antibacterial, antifungal qualities. The Ayurvedic technique of tongue scraping gently cleanses the tongue, one of the escape routes for toxins trying to leave your body. These toxins cause mucus and bacteria to build up at the base of the tongue, creating a white film. By gently scraping this coating off first thing in the morning, you avoid reabsorbing these toxins and ensure sweet breath. Another healthy Ayurvedic practice is known as "oil pulling." Oil pulling is simply rinsing the mouth with approximately one tablespoon of sesame oil or coconut oil, which reduces oral bacteria, soothes the gums and mouth tissue, and may reduce dental plaque. It's recommended to practice oil pulling in the morning on an empty stomach, gently swishing for fifteen to twenty seconds before spitting out the oil (it's important not to swallow the oil because it will accumulate toxins).

THE THROAT

It is through the amazing instrument we call our throat that we express ourselves. There are many things we can do to enhance and take care of the throat. Consume raw honey mixed with fresh-squeezed lemon juice to soothe the throat. Gargle with salt water to help clear throat infections. Massage your throat from time to time, as it is a common place to hold fear and is responsive to the touch of compassion. It is also the location of the fifth chakra, the purification chakra. By expressing ourselves and being mindful of not hiding things inside, but instead making it a priority to let them out (even on paper), we can stay clear. Other beautiful ways to care for the throat are through singing, reciting poetry, chanting, praying, and laughing … all wonderful for opening the throat and keeping it clear and vibrant.

THE NOSE

At the time of this writing, I've been traveling long distances and have come down with a major sinus infection, so it's time to take this area of the body seriously. I had always heard about the benefits of neti pots and nasal sprays but had basically denied these disciplines … but no longer! The yogis say we should breathe through our nose, not our mouth, as there is a natural air filter in the nostrils—our nose hairs. These help filter out dust, bugs, and other

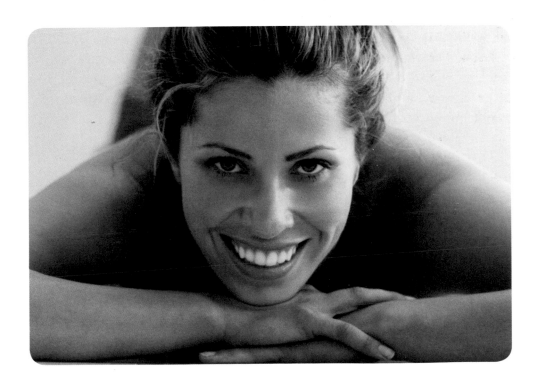

DAY SEVENTEEN TOOLKIT

unnecessary pollutants. For eons, the yogis have used the neti pot by filling it with warm water and noniodized salt (like Celtic sea salt), and pouring the water through one nostril and letting it gently drain out the other. This helps clear out the toxins and makes way for a cleaner air filter and easy breathing.

Yoga for Beauty Pose of the Day: *Triangle Pose*

Begin with your left leg forward, right foot back. Your back right foot is at a ninety-degree angle to your front left foot (heel to arch). Your legs are straight without being locked or hyperextended (try slightly bending the front knee). As you inhale, lift and lengthen the waist and engage the legs. As you exhale, reach forward with your front left arm and lengthen your torso while you bring your body into a gentle side stretch. Only go as far as you can keep your back straight, as if against an imaginary wall. Your shoulders move down away from your ears. Neck stays long as you reach your right arm up toward the sky. Stay for at least five breaths and then, on an inhale, bring your body back up. Repeat on the second side (aka the easy side).

Mantra of the Day:

I AM THE ONE
I HAVE BEEN
WAITING FOR.

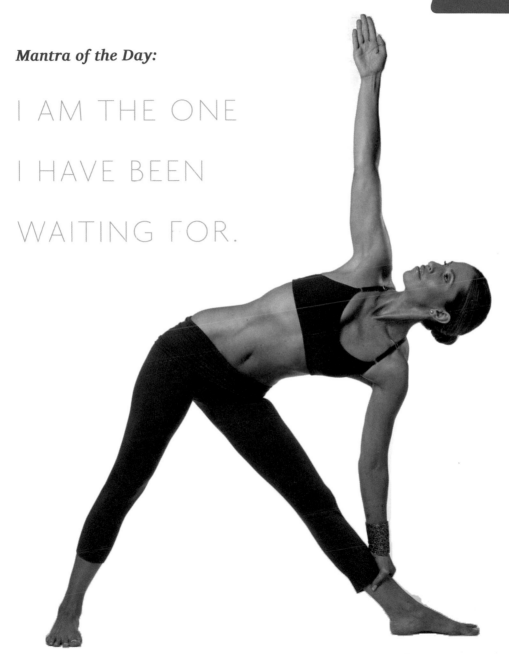

DAY EIGHTEEN SCHEDULE

7:00 AM DAWN GLOW TONIC
Start with the liver tonic of your choice
Enjoy a warm cup of mint, ginger, and honey tea.

8:00 AM BREAKFAST
Start the day with Energy Soup for long lasting energy (page 315)
Drink barley grass powder in water for extra-radiant skin

10:00 AM YOGA POSE OF THE DAY
Option: *Yoga for Beauty* or *ra'yoKa* Sequence of the Day
Option: Listen to a guided meditation or sit in meditation for fifteen minutes

12:00 NOON LUNCH
Magical Mermaid Soup (page 315)
Option: Raw blended dessert, like lemon meringue, but be sure to eat it first so it digests better.

1:00 PM SELF-TLC
Option: Practice conscious breathing (*pranayama*)
Option: Contemplate today's action step for Aligning with Your Ultimate Purpose

4:00 PM	DINNER	
	Recipe of the Day: Raw Prosperity Soup (page 317)	

6:00 PM	GET YOUR GLOW ON	
	Walking Meditation: Observe every bone as you move	

AS DESIRED	SNACKS & DESSERTS	
	Vanilla almond milk with a touch of cinnamon and raw honey	

7:00 PM	DUSK GLOW TONIC	
	Fresh coconut water	

SUPPLEMENTAL RECOMMENDATION

It's time to consider a near-future fast day or gallbladder cleanse. Journal about the things you might be craving at this point in your process. Refer to the Week Three Reflections on page 276 for writing prompts. Do this while sipping on some hot apple cider vinegar and lemon for a little alkalizing comfort.

DAY EIGHTEEN **TOOLKIT**

Virtue of the Day: *Diligence*

There are moments, and sometimes days, during any cleanse or fast when the process of physical detoxification (as well as the emotional and mental purging that takes place) can leave you feeling tired and unfocused. If you find yourself moving a little more slowly and feeling some laziness creep in, know that it will pass. You can also shift that energy by choosing one task to tend to today that you will give your full attention and care, even if only for a few minutes. Take ten to thirty minutes (or whatever amount of time feels right) and get something checked off your to-do list. For example, you could take fifteen minutes to diligently go through your email inbox and delete old emails. You may feel an upward rise in your energy as you persevere in getting some small action item completed.

Action Step of the Day: *Aligning with Your Ultimate Purpose*

Just as the seasons transition from winter to spring, our bodies also flow through various energetic cycles. By acknowledging our natural rhythms, we can tap into their intrinsic powers to become our healthiest and most beautiful selves.

According to Traditional Chinese Medicine, winter is associated with the Water element. Wet, flowing, surrendering, the seedbed of all life, the Water element represents the Kidney meridian (yin, feminine) and the Urinary-Bladder meridian (yang, masculine). The kidneys also store *jing*, our vital essence that serves as the root of yin and yang for the entire body. *Jing* is disturbed and depleted by the emotions of fear or paranoia.

In the spring, a time of birth and renewal, we see sprouts of green blossoming everywhere. Likewise, in our bodies energies and substances are also

RECIPE OF THE DAY: **RAW PROSPERITY SOUP**

This warming and lively soup is nourishing to kidneys, bladder, reproductive system, lungs, and creativity.

INGREDIENTS

- 1 cup chopped carrots
- 1½ cups coconut water (young Thai coconut)
- ½ cup coconut meat (young Thai coconut)
- 1 orange
- ½ cup walnuts or almonds (soaked and rinsed)
- 1 teaspoon ginger
- 1 teaspoon cinnamon
- 1 clove garlic (optional)
- 2 tablespoons raw honey, maple syrup, or a few dates (optional)

DIRECTIONS

Blend all of the ingredients until creamy. Before eating, bless your soup with: *I allow abundance and prosperity into my life.*

DAY EIGHTEEN **TOOLKIT**

brought to the surface, making it easier to detox. As we enlighten ourselves, we can embody the energy of eternal spring—associated with the Wood element, which is expressed in the body by our bones, joints, muscles, ligaments, tendons, and spine. The energy of Wood flows strongly through the Liver meridian (yin) and Gallbladder meridian (yang). Imbalance within the Wood element can manifest as anger, depression, indecisiveness, frustration, and stagnation. As we shift into spring, we awaken from our period of rest, entering into the exuberance of growth. This growth can be observed as the expansion of plant life, physical energy, and the creative action that spring tends to ignite. We transition from abstract and yielding Water to the tangible co-creative impulses of Wood.

You can flow through these changes with grace by adopting some of these simple and healthy habits:

SPRING CLEANSING
Detoxify the liver, kidneys, gallbladder, lungs, and intestines to remove wastes in your body. Get a fresh start daily with a Lemon Kick or herbal tea like nettles (high in iron and good for the kidneys), dandelion root (a marvelous liver tonic), and red clover (to purify the blood).

DRINK PLENTY OF PURE WATER
Essential for cleansing the body, especially through the kidneys and bladder.

THE KIDNEY RUB
A Taoist exercise, the Kidney Rub is performed on the backside of the body, right underneath the lowest ribs. Make a fist and rub up and down in a quick motion thirty-six times to nourish this vital area, which governs the health of your hair, as well as your passion and fearlessness in the world.

EXERCISE

Referencing what ancient Chinese philosophy refers to as the Tao, the nurturing of life requires that we stay as fluid and flexible as possible. While cleansing, stay in motion with restorative postures and activities, taking care not to remain still for too long (sedentary). For the sake of balance, also take care not to drive yourself to exhaustion by trying to perform overly strenuous or impossible tasks.

SAY GRACE

As we know, when allowed to go unchecked, stress can impair immune and metabolic functions. Yet one of the most potent stress relievers available is as simple as our own heartfelt words. Dr. Masaru Emoto's remarkable book *The Hidden Messages in Water* provides proof that thoughts and feelings indeed affect physical reality. Presenting the results of his experiments photographing three-dimensional crystals, Dr. Emoto shows what happens to the same water samples when exposed to a variety of written and spoken words, as well as music. Stunning photographs show how the water appears to change its "expression," forming into harmonic hexagonal shapes when given positive stimulus and producing misshapen/diseased images when given negative influences. So bless each sip of water with your daily mantra and go with the flow.

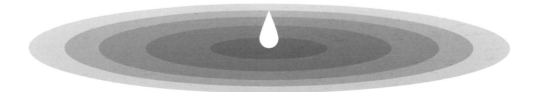

Water flows humbly to the lowest level. Nothing is more flexible and yielding than water. Yet for overcoming what is hard and strong, nothing surpasses it. —LAO TZU

DAY EIGHTEEN **TOOLKIT**

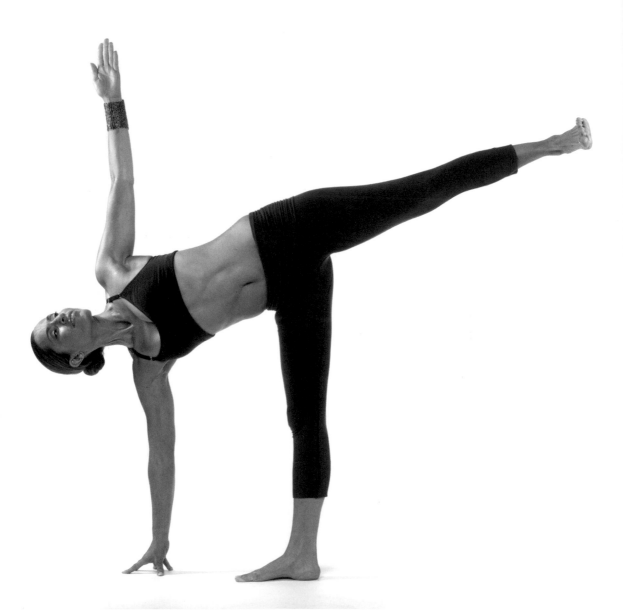

Yoga for Beauty Pose or ra'yoKa Sequence of the Day:
Half Moon Pose

Begin by standing tall with your feet together (Mountain Pose), and then step forward into a wide stance, leading with the right foot. Perform Extended Triangle Pose to the right, with your left hand on your left hip. Inhale as you bend your right knee, reaching your right hand onto the floor about six inches forward and an inch to the right. On an inhale, while grounding your right foot into the floor, straighten your right leg and lift your left leg back and parallel to the floor. Engage energetically through your left heel to keep your leg strong. Rotate your upper torso, opening at the side. For balance, steady your gaze and think "we go down to go up." Stay in this position for five to seven breaths. To release, lower your raised leg to the floor with an exhalation (returning to Extended Triangle), and then step back into Mountain Pose. Repeat the posture on your left for the same length of time. *ra'yoKa* variation: to increase stamina and focus, simply return to standing Mountain Pose up to ten times, remembering to breathe and use your hand as little as possible.

Mantra of the Day:

IF NOT NOW, THEN WHEN WILL I LET MY TRUE AND DIVINE NATURE BE MY OFFERING?

DAY NINETEEN SCHEDULE

7:00 AM DAWN GLOW TONIC
Start with the liver tonic of your choice
Try a cup of warm water with a touch of cacao powder and vanilla and a splash of fresh almond milk

8:00 AM BREAKFAST
A Latin American: blend a papaya with raw honey and cinnamon

10:00 AM YOGA POSE OF THE DAY
Option: *Yoga for Beauty* Pose of the Day
Option: Sprinting at a nearby park

12:00 NOON LUNCH
Blend miso in gently warmed water with seaweed, nut cheese (perhaps some kelp noodles for texture), warm and spice to taste
Option: Energy Soup (page 315)
Option: Smashed banana with Celtic sea salt, honey, and cinnamon

1:00 PM SELF-TLC
Option: Give yourself a mini-facial treatment. See Day Twenty "Action Step of the Day" on page 258 for facial ideas and inspiration.
Option: Contemplate today's action step for Aligning with Your Ultimate Purpose

DAY **19** ★

| 4:00 PM | DINNER |
| | Recipe of the Day: Live Divine Chocolate Maca Shake (page 335) |

6:00 PM	GET YOUR GLOW ON
	Try a *ra'yoKa* download, maybe level Blue (Therapeutics) or Level Orange for detox
	Option: Brush your hair with rosemary oil and jojoba

| AS DESIRED | SNACKS & DESSERTS |
| | Smashed avocado with a pinch of Celtic sea salt and either cumin or cayenne |

| 7:00 PM | DUSK GLOW TONIC |
| | ACV Tonic with lemon and raw honey (page 330) |

SUPPLEMENTAL RECOMMENDATION

Consider doing a warm castor oil compress on your liver tonight. Visualize any old and stuck emotions being released from your liver and body as you continue on with your renewing cleanse. Love yourself enough to pay attention to your vital organs; they do so much for us, but we rarely give back.

Castor Oil Compress

ITEMS:
A hot water bottle/bag
Linen cloth
Castor oil
Hand towel
Large towel

DIRECTIONS: Soak the linen cloth in the castor oil and place on your liver area, located right below the front ribs on the right side of the body. Place the hand towel on top of the linen cloth, then the hot water bottle, and then cover it with the larger towel to keep in the warmth and protect things from getting all oily. Visualize the liver bathed in radiant yellow and healed with this new light. If necessary, reheat the water.

DAY NINETEEN **TOOLKIT**

Virtue of the Day: *Chastity*

Chastity is the kind of word that conjures images of bygone eras, times when sexual repression was all the rage. However, the true energy of chastity is transformational, not repressive. When we abstain from something mindfully and for the purpose of cultivating an inner state of meditation, we are, in essence, practicing chastity. On this fifth day of Week Three, as you continue to abstain from toxins that may have resulted from bad relationship choices or internal wounds, notice the internal "cleanness" that comes from taking in living, blended foods.

Action Step of the Day: *Aligning with Your Ultimate Purpose*

The heart is the sacred symbol of the pulse of life. When we close down in an attempt to protect our hearts, we can experience depression, anxiety, and loneliness, and find ourselves faced with life-threatening ailments such as heart disease. When we choose to keep an open heart, no matter how much heartache we've gone through, the whole world opens itself to us.

For every one of us, our hearts intimately know our ultimate purpose and will guide us in that direction every time we're willing to listen. The following suggestions are simple and practical ways to care for your heart today—to soothe it, listen to its whispers, and give it the support it needs:

PHYSICAL ALIGNMENT
Keeping your shoulders integrated and in alignment helps the chest area and heart remain available and open. Simply draw them back, and down to support the chest opening forward.

DAY 19

RECIPE OF THE DAY: **LIVE DIVINE CHOCOLATE MACA SHAKE**

A heart-opening and hormone-enhancing celebration in a glass.

INGREDIENTS

- ¼ cup Brazil nuts (soaked and rinsed) or other raw nuts
- 1 ripe avocado
- 1 semi-frozen banana
- 2 tablespoons raw honey or maple syrup (optional)
- 1 cup Brazil nut milk (option: almond or coconut milk, or pure water)
- 2 to 3 tablespoons raw cacao powder
- 1 tablespoon bee pollen (optional)
- 1 tablespoon maca powder
- 1 teaspoon cinnamon powder
- ½ teaspoon Celtic sea salt

DIRECTIONS

Blend all the ingredients until smooth. Add cold or room-temperature water if needed to adjust to desired thickness (but do not add warm water or heat this recipe). *Option: Spice it up by adding Living Libations Immune Illume Hotberry.*

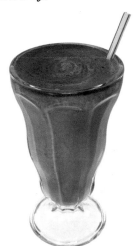

DAY NINETEEN **TOOLKIT**

Yoga for Beauty Sequence of the Day: *Jump-Throughs*

In yoga, there are different ways to move from posture to posture. Use this posture to cultivate awareness through each movement you make. Start in Downward-Facing Dog; press down evenly through your palms and all five fingers. On your exhale, lift up through your core. You must look forward beyond any obstacles. As your heart and head have intention, your feet will follow, so gracefully jump your feet through and beyond your arms. Move your feet through your hands and come to a seated position. End in Dandasana (Seated Stick Pose). Let go of the last moment, whether you achieved it or not, and breathe.

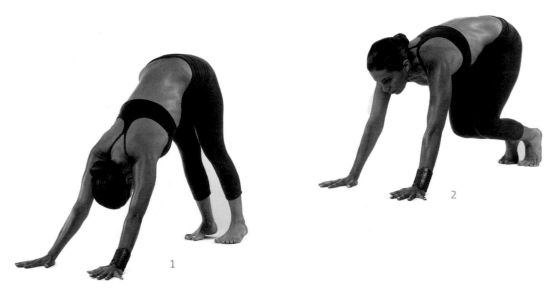

Practice ... and all is coming. —SRI K. PATABHI JOIS

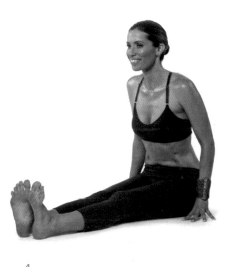

1

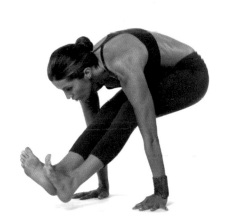

3

Mantra of the Day:

I SURRENDER IN DEVOTION

TO THE MOTION

AND I CELEBRATE

AS I CREATE.

DAY TWENTY SCHEDULE

7:00 AM DAWN GLOW TONIC
Start with the liver tonic of your choice
Fresh-squeezed watermelon (or fruit in season) and
nettles or mint

8:00 AM BREAKFAST
Juice—celery, cucumber, tomato, and lemon. Make a lot
and drink all day. Add kale and ginger if you like. Consider
fasting and drinking only juices today.

10:00 AM YOGA POSE OF THE DAY
Option: *Yoga for Beauty* Pose of the Day
Option: Pop in *Yoga for Beauty: Dawn* DVD

12:00 NOON LUNCH
Continue drinking the juice you made for breakfast
or make more

1:00 PM SELF-TLC
Option: Meditate on today's mantra
Option: Contemplate today's action step for Aligning with
Your Ultimate Purpose

DAY **20** ★

4:00 PM	DINNER
	Recipe of the Day: Mystic Mango Smoothie (page 335)
	Option: More juice!

6:00 PM	GET YOUR GLOW ON
	Consider meditating and chanting devotional music or mantras for inner peace and clarity.

AS DESIRED	SNACKS & DESSERTS
	Drink more fresh juice: add olive oil and a pinch of salt for more substance

7:00 PM	DUSK GLOW TONIC
	Ginger, mint, and lemon tea

SUPPLEMENTAL RECOMMENDATION

Last chance: If you haven't already tried an enema or colonic, I am recommending it. You don't want to wait until you've completed the cleanse to try it, as it will be less comfortable. It's much better now when things are moving and flowing and detoxification is under way.

DAY TWENTY **TOOLKIT**

Virtue of the Day: *Soberness*

You are almost there! You have arrived at Day Twenty of the cleanse. See how far a blender and a strong commitment can take you?! Today, acknowledge the self-discipline you employed to get to this point in the process. Notice the paradox that you have been willing to play with—discovering that beauty and indulgence can coexist. There is a beautiful soberness that comes from cleaning out the body and feeding it high-energy foods, an alertness that allows us to see through the illusion of things. Take note of what you see today through your sober eyes.

Action Step of the Day: *Aligning with Your Ultimate Purpose*

Today is dedicated to gaining clarity of vision (both inner and outer) and caring for the eyes and face that allow us to meet the world anew each day. The following treatments and activities will restore balance, strength, and beauty, especially when incorporated on a consistent basis:

The forehead center, or "the third eye," is the gateway of intuition. It is the home of the sixth chakra, the chakra of knowing and perceiving. It's through this area that deep relaxation can be induced. In Ayurveda, there is a luxurious treatment called *shirodhara,* in which warm oil is slowly poured over the forehead for a thirty-minute period—easily melting away body tension and mental noise. If you haven't experienced this healing treat, I highly recommend it.

THE EYES

Did you know that having "bags under the eyes" can be a sign that the kidneys are under stress? One way to support the kidneys and clear puffy eyes is to drink a quart of nettle tea. Also, examine the foods you're eating, because you

RECIPE OF THE DAY: **MYSTIC MANGO SMOOTHIE**

A luscious antioxidant blend for the nourishment of eyes, skin, and soul.

INGREDIENTS

- ¾ cup fresh (preferred) or frozen blackberries
- 1 mango, pitted and chopped
- ⅛ cup goji berries
- ¼ cup pomegranate juice or coconut water (pure water is good too)
- 1 tablespoon cacao or coconut butter
- 1 tablespoon royal jelly or bee pollen
- 1 teaspoon maca powder (optional)

DIRECTIONS

Combine all ingredients, blend until smooth, and serve.

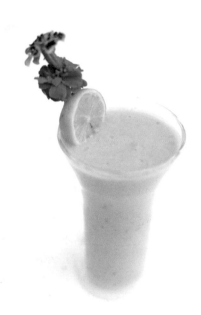

DAY TWENTY **TOOLKIT**

may have food allergies or sensitivities. Eyes also correspond to the liver. The forehead corresponds to the small intestines, the cheeks correspond to the lungs, and the chin corresponds to the reproductive area. We are given clues as to what areas may be out of balance. Notice what changes you are seeing in your face as you proceed through the days of the cleanse. The increase in water and clean foods is undoubtedly showing in your amazing face.

EYE EXERCISES

Exercising your eyes regularly can improve your vision and balance the hemispheres of your brain. Look side to side, up and down, and diagonally. Roll your eyes halfway in each direction, and then in full circles in both directions.

TREATMENTS FOR THE FACE

Facials are one of my favorite beauty rituals. Do it yourself or have someone do it for you. Here are a few self-care tips for facial radiance:

Clean your face with a good, nonchemical face wash such as Josie Maran Argan Cleansing Oil, free of mineral oils, synthetic colors, fragrances, or preservatives. Use a gentle scrub to exfoliate dead skin cells if your face is not overly sensitive.

Massage your face with clarifying oils to moisturize the skin, and then wash again to improve circulation.

Steam your face over a pot of hot water, adding purifying herbs such as rosemary and lavender. Or use towels soaked in hot water to soften and open your skin, applying for approximately twenty minutes. Then with clean hands, and two tissues to cover your fingers completely, remove debris from any clogged pores.

For nourishing masks, try some of the following: yogurt or acidophilus mixed with a few of drops of lavender essential oil; a mashed-up and moisturizing avocado; or a freshly blended papaya (with its enzymes for gently digesting dead skin cells). Aloe is soothing but can be a bit drying unless mixed with other moisturizing ingredients. Mud can also be too drying for delicate facial skin, although I do love Aztec Secret Indian Healing Clay. For a super fresh glow, take the peel of whatever fruit you used for your daily smoothie and rub it on a clean face. Wait for twenty minutes and then rinse off and use a toner. For a great DIY revitalizing mask, combine one eighth cup coconut kefir, Josie Maran Pure Argan Oil, and one tablespoon raw honey. Apply to your face, relax for ten minutes, then remove it. Apple cider vinegar can be dabbed onto zits and works amazingly well. Always finish your cleansing with a splash of cold water to tighten the pores. And for increasing your superstar glow, a spray of rose water before applying your moisturizer can be wonderful.

FACIAL EXERCISES

Tension causes the lines and rigidity that age us. One great way to keep the face from freezing into one position is to move the jaw from side to side and in and out, which helps melt that jaw tension away. Another tension reliever is to stick out your tongue and stretch your mouth open wide. Also, smiling uses fewer muscles than frowning, so go back and forth between the two exercises to relieve tension and relax the muscles.

FACIAL ACUPRESSURE

While watching your favorite television show or relaxing on your couch, press your cheeks, temples, forehead, chin, and hairline. This will promote the circulation of oxygen, blood, and lymph, while simultaneously stimulating important acupressure points (you don't even have to know where they are to benefit from this!). In some circles this is called the "acupressure facelift" and can result in noticeable benefits when done regularly. *Side note for a happy face: Remember that it is best to sleep on your back. Sleeping with your face smashed into a pillow can result in permanent facial lines.*

DAY TWENTY **TOOLKIT**

Yoga for Beauty Pose of the Day: Bow Pose

Modern lifestyles that keep us at our desks and seated in cars contribute to abdominal stagnation, which can impair digestion and lymphatic flow through our core. This torso-lengthening pose increases blood flow and supports our organs. *Dhanurasana* in Sanskrit (*dhanu* means bow), this pose resembles an archer's bow. Begin by lying on your belly with your hands alongside your torso, palms up. (You can lie on a folded blanket for padding if needed.) Exhale and bend your knees, bringing your heels as close as you can to your buttocks. Reach back with your hands and take hold of your ankles (optional adjustment: use a strap to wrap around the ankles to assist in reaching the hands back). Keep your knees no more than hip-width apart (if you're flexible) for the duration of the pose to protect the back. Inhale and pull your heels up away from your buttocks as you lift your thighs away from the floor. Keeping your back muscles supple, raise your chest and let the head follow, allowing your tailbone to be heavy toward the floor. If this is a good stretch already, stay here for a few easy breaths, exhale and release down, enjoying the energy just cultivated in the body. For advanced practitioners, when you repeat, continue lifting your heels and thighs higher. Keep your neck long, and with the strength of your legs, open that area of your body called your heart. Release as you exhale, and repeat twice more. Please take five to ten breaths each round.

Mantra of the Day:

I BREATHE, BELIEVE, AND RECEIVE FROM MY HEART.

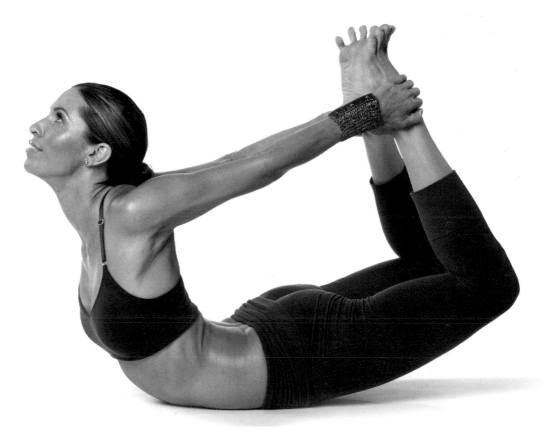

IN GRATITUDE IS WHERE I START.

DAY TWENTY-ONE **SCHEDULE**

7:00 AM	DAWN GLOW TONIC
	Hot Apple Cider Tea (page 334)
8:00 AM	BREAKFAST
	Live Chocolate Shake (page 334)
	Option: 1 bowl of Chia Pudding (page 326) with raw honey, cinnamon, and almond milk
10:00 AM	YOGA POSE OF THE DAY
	Option: *Yoga for Beauty* Pose of the Day
	Option: Walk in nature and remember to take in the sounds and sights ... and smell the flowers
12:00 NOON	LUNCH
	Recipe of the Day: Deva in Seva Harmony Tonic (page 333)
1:00 PM	SELF-TLC
	Option: Journal about what you've experienced over the past three weeks; do this outside as you observe the birds and bees.
	Option: Contemplate today's action step for Aligning with Your Ultimate Purpose

| 4:00 PM | DINNER |
| | Blend up whatever version of Energy Soup you most enjoy (page 315) |

| 6:00 PM | GET YOUR GLOW ON |
| | Try *Yoga for Beauty: Dusk* or Level Purple *ra'yoKa* downloads. |

| AS DESIRED | SNACKS & DESSERTS |
| | Fresh pressed juice such as pinapple-mint or strawberry-lemon |

| 7:00 PM | DUSK GLOW TONIC |
| | Ginger tea with raw honey, lemon, and a splash of apple cider vinegar |

SUPPLMENTAL RECOMMENDATION

Consider flushing out the blood by taking a supplement that stimulates circulation, like cayenne, garlic, or if you're comfortable with it, the amazing niacin (vitamin B3). Feel the blood flow and fat melt as your body temperature rises. Placing orange oil in the bath can get your circulation flowing as well.

DAY TWENTY-ONE TOOLKIT

Virtue of the Day: *Harmony*

Prior to starting the twenty-one-day cleanse, you may have been experiencing the discord that comes from eating overly processed foods, or from sheer over-consumption of habits or foods that distribute pollutants throughout the system. On this final day of Week Three, as you listen to the whirling musicality of your blender again today, sense the harmony you have invited into your body and life over the past twenty days. Take time to consciously notice if and where you feel more connected to yourself, your loved ones, your work, and the world around you.

Action Step of the Day: *Aligning with Your Ultimate Purpose*

Congratulations on reaching the final day of *The 21-Day SuperStar Cleanse!* The past three weeks have been a period of release and renewal. In addition to physical changes, you have released limiting patterns and embraced new ones that support and promote your optimal well-being. All of this movement could be summarized as a process of healing, aligning, and becoming more alive.

As you journey onward as your *refreshed* self, you may be freshly inspired to integrate new practices as part of a more holistic lifestyle, one that honors your interconnectedness with other people and our living planet.

The following practical habits and observances can be incorporated by each one of us to help stoke the warm fires of our communal life together on this exquisite earth.

RECIPE OF THE DAY: **DEVA IN SEVA HARMONY TONIC**

In Sanskrit, *Deva* means divine being and *Seva* is the spirit of selfless service. This tonic offers a toast to both of these aspects within you.

INGREDIENTS

- 1 to 2 apples
- 1 beet
- ¼ cup chopped or shredded purple cabbage
- 1-inch piece daikon radish
- 1-inch piece ginger
- 1 handful blackberries and/or grapes (as in season)
- 1 teaspoon gotu kola (optional)

DIRECTIONS

1. Juice all of the ingredients.
2. Stir in gotu kola or your favorite superfood supplements.

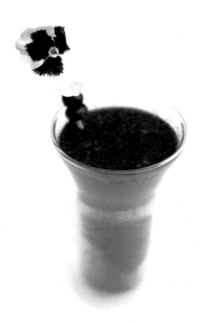

DAY TWENTY-ONE **TOOLKIT**

Mindful Eating: Bring a sense of gratitude and awareness into every meal

- Reflect on the origins of your food. Is it organic? Local? From a company that is committed to sustainable practices?

- Delight in every bite. As you avoid distractions while you eat (like watching TV, surfing the Internet, or driving), chew thoroughly and savor the flavors.

- Avoid sensory "junk" food. What we consume includes what we see, read, hear, feel, think, and say. What kind of sensory input does your highest self desire?

- Be Here Now … as the old saying goes. Cultivate awareness and presence as you prepare, serve, and eat your meals. Everyday tasks can be a nurturing meditation. Another way to be in the present is to choose produce that's in the present—go seasonal!

- Share your meals. Connect with loved ones by cooking and eating together. Try a new recipe with friends or surprise someone with a homemade treat. In some cultures, communities dine together at one big table and take turns spoon-feeding each other rather than everyone eating for themselves. By eating in this way, everyone consumes half as much yet becomes twice as full.

- Give thanks. Again, we come back to gratitude and deep appreciation. Pausing to bring your awareness to the blessings and nourishment you are about to receive brings greater satisfaction and a multidimensional sense of fullness from smaller portions.

Conscious Consumption: Harvesting abundance on a finite planet

- Eat sustainably. Along with eating more organic, local, and seasonal foods, consider eating lower on the food chain for the benefit of all (less meat, more plants). When you can, learn about the practice of permaculture.

- Conserve energy. Unplug unused appliances, wash clothes in cold water, use a clothesline or drying rack, and turn the lights down low earlier in the evenings.

- Save water. Plant drought-tolerant and native plants, take shorter showers, and use low-flow appliances.

- Let off the gas. Walk or bike, carpool, telecommute, drive electric and hybrid cars.

- Do it yourself. The average person uses more than ten personal care products per day, many of which are replaced every month. Experiment with making some of your own cleaning supplies, toiletries, and cosmetics. Not only will this reduce the buildup of wasteful packaging, you might create some irresistible recipes that you love using.

- Invest in the future. As you know, many of our purchases soon end up in ever-growing landfills. Remember to reduce, reuse, and recycle. Try second-hand products from garage sales, thrift stores, or online. Borrow from the library. Share tools and appliances with loved ones and neighbors. Buy in bulk. And invest in long-lasting, quality products.

DAY TWENTY-ONE **TOOLKIT**

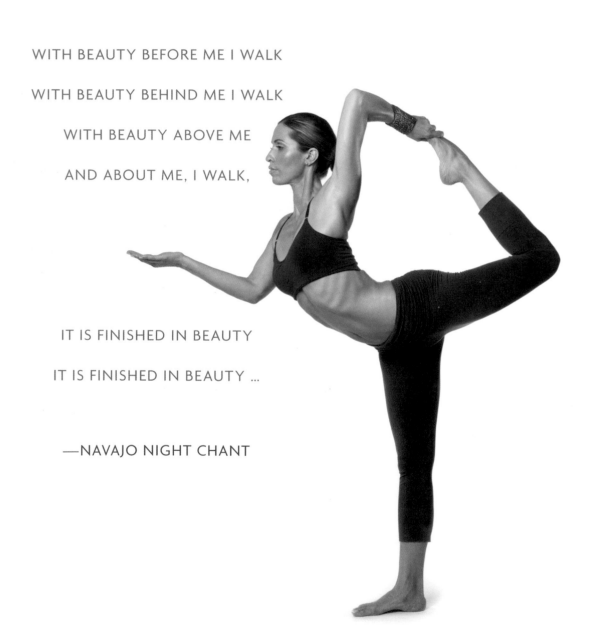

WITH BEAUTY BEFORE ME I WALK

WITH BEAUTY BEHIND ME I WALK

WITH BEAUTY ABOVE ME

AND ABOUT ME, I WALK,

IT IS FINISHED IN BEAUTY

IT IS FINISHED IN BEAUTY ...

—NAVAJO NIGHT CHANT

Yoga Pose of the Day: *Dancer's Pose*

Begin by standing straight with your legs together and toes spread (Mountain Pose). Shift your weight to your right leg as you bend your left leg up behind you. Maintain balance as you reach back to grasp your left ankle with your left hand and slightly pull your leg toward the back hip to release the psoas muscle (be careful not to bend your leg back too far or too quickly). Keep breathing as you press down through your standing leg, mindful to keep your spine straight and erect. Move down and back to feel gravity anchoring and aligning you. Using the mechanics of lifting, rise up to create a deeper back bend while maintaining a broad lower back. As we inhale, we find more space. As we exhale we choose more strength. Maintain balance in Dancer's Pose for five to ten breaths. Breathe deeply as you allow the pose to help cultivate space in your legs, thighs, hips, abdomen, spine, chest, and shoulders. Then relax your right arm as you let go of your left ankle to return to standing. After a brief rest, repeat the pose on your other side for an equal duration of time.

Mantra of the Day:

MY PATH IS MADE BY WALKING ON IT.

ILLUMINATIONS
week three

With a fresh tea, a pressed juice, or perhaps a Live Chocolate Shake in hand, enjoy the following section designed to deepen your understanding of the cleanse process and expand your level of inspiration.

Fasting from Toxins

"Fasting" can mean a multitude of different things. Fasting might refer to the consumption of a strictly plant-based diet in its most natural form (uncooked and unadulterated), an all-fruit diet, an all-blended foods diet (smoothies and soups), the consumption of fresh juices only, or in the most disciplined or austere terms, fasting with water only—or on frankincense and myrrh as holy men were said to have done.

Throughout time, spiritual leaders including Moses, Jesus, Mohammed, Buddha, and Gandhi have fasted for spiritual illumination and health. Plato, Socrates, and Hippocrates credited fasting with mental clarity and longevity. And in more recent times, enlightened physicians such Albert Schweitzer, Benjamin Spock, and Deepak Chopra have all agreed that fasting is one of the most neglected yet powerful healing techniques available to us. Some religious observations ask for fasting or abstaining from certain foods as well.

With so many powerful endorsements of fasting, it's a wonder we don't fast more often. However, there is truly no time like the present to discover its transformative capabilities.

BENEFITS OF FASTING

To name just a few …

- Increases energy
- Accelerates healing
- Gives our digestive systems a break
- Boosts metabolism
- Enhances immunity
- Releases excess toxins or accumulated fat from the body
- Weight loss
- Increases flexibility
- Clear complexion
- Shining eyes
- Relaxation and unraveling of tension in the body
- Deep, restful sleep
- Mental clarity
- Heals disease while resting and rejuvenating the immune system
- Positively affects ailments like heart disease, asthma, cancer, bronchitis, obesity, immune disorders, hypertension, arthritis, ulcers, and toxicity of any kind
- Moves us toward a complete regeneration of our bodies
- Longevity
- Unleashes creativity
- Increases awareness and insight
- Enhances ability to meditate and/or focus
- Divine inspiration

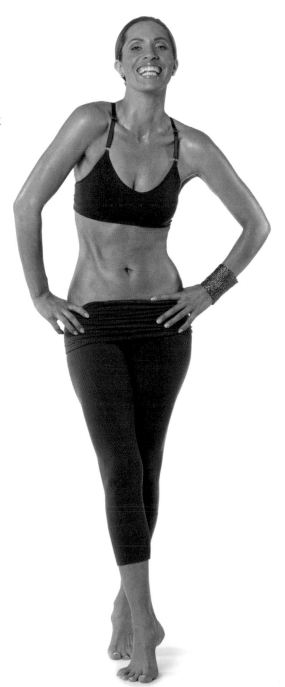

SUPERSTAR SKIN
finding your head-to-toe glow

One of the fantastic outcomes of cleansing and fasting from toxins for just about everyone is healthier, happier, and more beautiful skin. Our skin is governed by the health of our lungs and large intestines. So you may have noticed that eating foods and engaging in activities that support those magnificent organ systems show up very quickly in your skin.

The following tips can be added to your growing knowledge base of how to maintain your superstar glow for the rest of your life:

- Breathe deeply
- Drink plenty of cleansing water *(a mantra always worth repeating)*
- Enjoy avocados, seaweed, and olives to maintain or rebuild collagen
- Eat radishes, cucumbers, and greens for their stockpile of healthy minerals
- Include carrots, sweet potatoes, and squash to keep the skin resistant to infection
- Use quality multipurpose skin care products like Living Libations Seabuckthorn Best Skin Ever

The Beauty Bath: *At-home hydrotherapy for your body's overall glow*

For soft, glowing skin, try a dry-brush skin massage. This is excellent to do before getting into the shower or bath. It strengthens the immune system, improves circulation, moves lymphatic congestion, and exfoliates the dead cells. Simply use a dry brush all over your body (arms, legs, torso, and back, if you have a long-handled body brush) and gently massage the skin in a circular motion toward your heart.

Using a good salt, sugar, or loofah scrub in the shower is similar to a dry-brush skin massage, and will also leave your skin feeling super soft.

Steam baths are another great treatment. They open your pores, are great for your skin, and are beneficial for people with congested lungs or breathing problems.

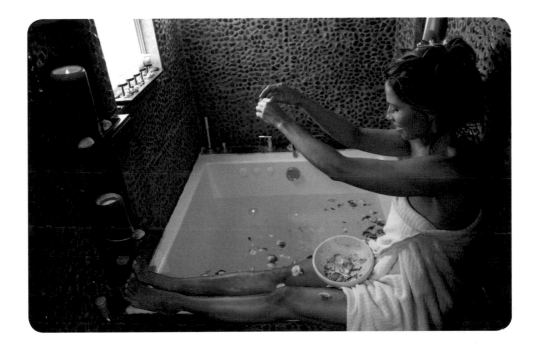

Add essential oils such as eucalyptus or bergamot to enhance the healing qualities of a steam bath. I personally prefer dry saunas and hot herbal baths for their warming qualities, where I can feel myself sweat and mindfully let go.

It is a tradition in many cultures to end a shower with cold water. It is refreshing and invigorating, and helps close and reduce the pores.

It is best to moisturize your skin when it is still slightly damp from your hydrotherapy session. As always, with facial moisturizer or body lotions, avoid mineral oils, synthetic fragrances, and dyes. Try Josie Maran Argon Oil Body Butter or coconut oil to stay on the natural side. Everything we put on our skin is absorbed through our cells. With certain lotions you can add essential oils. My favorites are rose, vanilla, and ylang ylang.

For more beautifying practices: See the Day Twenty Toolkit *on page 258 for suggestions on at-home facials, and visit the* 28 Beauty Rituals *section on page 370.*

REFLECTIONS
discovering yourself anew

As you have done in Weeks One and Two, continue to utilize your journal (or computer) for translating some of your new-felt experience into words. There is something special that happens when we allow our unique inner experience to flow through our pen and out on to paper. Sometimes unexpected clarity comes, a secret feeling or thought sees the light of day, or a private dream is proclaimed. At other times, it simply helps document our process in the simplest of ways—what we ate, what we drank, how much we weighed this morning, how it felt to take that yoga class, and what we plan to do tomorrow. So use your journaling time this week with the greatest of freedom, knowing that the blank page is all your own, here for the purpose of serving your journey of discovery and radiant wellness. The following questions can be useful in that process:

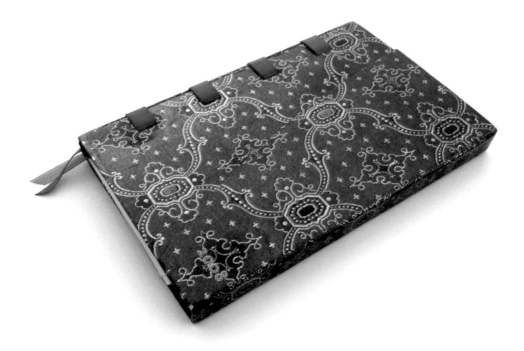

1. How has adding live, blended foods to your diet impacted your body this week? How has it made you feel? Any new sensations? Did you notice any changes in your digestion?

2. Did you experience mild or strong cravings? Were these cravings for certain foods, feelings, relationships, places, or activities?

3. What moods and emotions did you experience? Were you able to identify or name your emotions? And were you able to be present with those emotions?

4. Were you aware of any limiting thoughts or beliefs this week?

5. How easy or challenging was it to follow through with this week's recommendations and guidelines?

6. Which recipes, action steps, or tips did you incorporate? And how did it feel to increase your self-care?

7. How did it feel to exercise this week? Did you notice areas where you were more flexible? Have any areas of tension decreased?

8. Have your sleep patterns changed? Did you sleep less or more?

9. If you wanted to go—or actually went—off track, what were the triggers or common tipping points for you?

10. How connected do you feel right now with your higher purpose?

this is the hour

A POETIC VISUALIZATION

The following visualization is offered as a meditation on the light within you. It is an extended mantra that will serve you as a bridge from the three-week cleanse to reentering your life. Light a candle, find a comfortable and quiet place to read and reflect, and allow these words to remind you of your sacred wholeness.

From the center of my body
Like the sun, I inhale and I breathe out through rays into what's around
From the periphery of my being I exhale and connect more deeply to my core
Listening to my inner being and what I am truly here for

The bright light of my solar plexus
Inhale, expanding into the 72,000 pathways to my skin
I look for dark and shine light there
Then, exhale, travel back to the source where I began
And start again.

I seek out noises, shadows, triggers, wounds, and injuries
And ride the breath of clearing energy
To the surface of all I show
To find all that is within me and what I need to let go
I expand light on my inhale as I observe all that I don't even know

As I Inhale to expand
And exhale to contract
Only occasionally looking back
To find the teaching ... that I may be holding
To understand the root of where I am unfolding
To see which glitch on what hard drive may be affecting
My every manifestation in life,
But also my physical structure, and today's back bends or handstands.

The *sushumna* rises up through the center of the spine
The ray of light that helps us live, connect, and be guided purely by what's divine.
Connection to our pure perfection
I open and find
And the outcome is the enhancement of the shine.

The left side is the feminine
The right side is the masculine
The left receives
While the right one gives
Are they communicating?
Are they living respectfully in harmony with awareness ...
to one another?

The right side roots down
Deep into the ground
The spirals crossing and moving
Until balance is what is found
And I continue to listen to the breath
For where the inhale ends and the exhale begins ...
My being attunes to the unspoken silence that is beyond sound.

We know that the element of the core is fire
With this central flame ignited we will go higher
We embody who we really are
Solar beings, vehicles of light like each star
This is the hour
That we can remember

As the planets align
So does our soul
As we do the inner work
We become whole.

As simple as each breath
When we get out of our way
That infinite place that breathes us
The place beyond this dimension that we must trust
Beyond fear, doubt, gluttony, or lust
There is a place that awaits us that is a must

Where clarity and connection are strong
and the bridge of light becomes our song
This place is our birthright
it's there for us to take flight
and be

All that we've waited for is here
we just had to become clear
The work is and always was inside
all we must do is decide

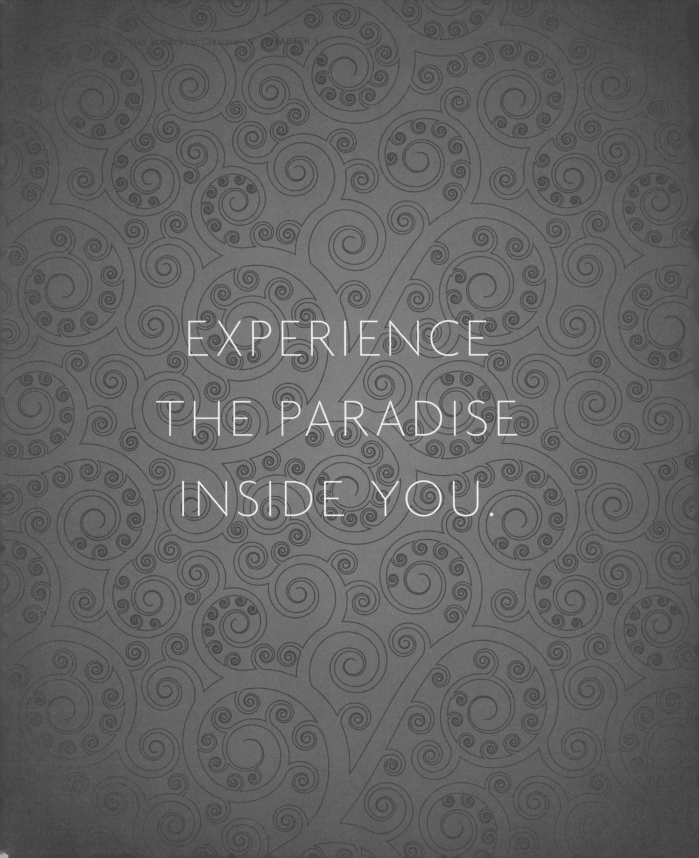

EXPERIENCE
THE PARADISE
INSIDE YOU.

REENTERING THE WORLD: INTEGRATION AND PLANNING

Although *The 21-Day SuperStar Cleanse* program is designed to fit into your daily life, exactly where you are, my hope is that you feel as though you have taken a vacation over the past three weeks—an inner vacation, like time spent in Hawaii, where your senses are awakened and your spirit is revived. I hope you can feel greater openness and vibrancy. Perhaps you can feel the soft trade winds of your dreams and desires caressing you, reminding you of why taking good care of yourself matters. A living foods cleanse has a way of doing this, a way of giving us the experience of the paradise that can be ours on the inside.

You know the feeling when you're returning from a vacation and you resolve not to lose the wellness and equanimity you found while you were away? It's the "How can I keep Hawaii with me?" moment. That is what this time is all about—discovering simple ways to bring some of the elements of your cleanse experience into your normal routine. This is your period of reintegration and easing back into your usual flow, but with new tools and practices to support your continual unfolding. As you look back over the past three weeks and ahead toward your future, ask yourself, "What can I keep from this experience? What can I carry with me?" As we will explore in the pages ahead, in addition to certain activities you might choose to make an ongoing part of your life (making kale salad, journaling, yoga, or collaging), this week is a great time to consider how you can continue with healing foods and lifestyle additions that work for you.

Whether you have been eating mainly blended foods over the past week, or have stayed with a clean vegan diet (even if just barely), or supplemented it with juices and superfoods, you have essentially been on a fast from toxins. How you reenter your regular life today and over the next week is just as important as (if not more important than) the cleanse itself. I've seen people undermine the benefits of their cleanse by not resolving it properly, so I am excited to outline a path of reintegration that you can tailor to your liking. After this period of digestive rest, your body needs to be gradually initiated into what will become your normal behaviors of eating (your "new normal"). To avoid shocking your freshly alleviated system with an onslaught of radical components, be careful to not binge on foods that your shiny new system will perceive as poison. Following a cleanse, your body is more sensitized to toxic substances that invade its pure temple. Similar to how you might warm up before exercising to help prevent injury, now is a time to honor your intestinal repose and gently restore your consumption as you would tenderly rouse a child from a nap.

One of the most important ways to do this is to eat slowly and chew your food thoroughly in order to acclimate your body to receiving more solid and, eventually, cooked foods. To assist in the transition, continue with fresh juices, morning Liver Kicks, superfood smoothies, raw or warmed soups, and vibrant salads. Remember: it's not an all-or-nothing proposition; you don't have to let yourself go too much. Like many of my friends, clients, and cleanse participants, you might find that incorporating energizing foods and drinks becomes a way of life. The main objective is to find and create a whole foods lifestyle that truly works for you, so feel free to taste and enjoy—explore as your conscience guides you, without neglecting the gems of the superstar discipline that brought you to your newfound state of health.

Before sending you off into the detailed portion of this chapter, I would like to shine a bright light on the three keys that I know can result in a successful 365-day way of life:

1. Follow the principles of food combining that are outlined in this chapter.
2. Become increasingly conscious of where your food comes (the farm, the importer, the company, the people, and their practices).
3. Tune in to each bite as a three-dimensional experience, one where beauty, health, and indulgence coexist.

Now you are ready to plan your strategy for a successful transition. As you do this, let yourself imagine how you can apply the benefits of this cleanse to a successful regime and, over time, turn them into 365 days a year that include an abundance of health-giving foods. Each organ has its season of healing and living in a life of normal stresses, festivities, excuses, and indulgences; eating even a semihealthy diet can still lead to a sluggish system if we don't pay our beings and bodies the special attention they deserve. So continue tuning back into this program seasonally (join an interactive, global, virtual program if you choose), as life permits.

RECOMMENDED TRANSITION
week four

DAY 22

Now it's time to devote an additional week to integrating your experience. On this first day of reentry, start your morning with a Liver Kick tonic or a glass of pure water with apple cider vinegar and raw honey. Continue hydrating and nourishing your body with enzyme-rich foods that encourage and support the flow you have cultivated these past three weeks. Begin introducing solid foods by eating a piece of fruit, a small salad with avocado (chewed completely), and/or a raw and slightly warmed soup. Also, continue juicing throughout the day.

DAY 23

On the second day, follow the same guidelines as yesterday, but with a slight increase in portion sizes. Adding flaxseeds and fruits like figs, raisins, or prunes soaked in pure water will help stimulate the bowels and assist your body in transitioning to solid foods.

DAY 24

Today, build on the second day. Continue to re-culture your system and introduce modest quantities of foods such as sprouts, fermented foods (coconut kefir, vegan yogurt, sauerkraut, seed cheese), and nut butters. If you prefer, try cooked whole grain (quinoa, millet, wild rice, amaranth, or buckwheat), but preferably, soak the grains first overnight with ample water and rinse. Chew all foods well and hydrate between meals with plenty of fresh juice, pure water, and herbal tea.

DAY 25

On this fourth of reentering, return to the guidelines and recipes of Week Two, being mindful not to overeat to the point of feeling full.

DAYS 26 TO 28

Transition back to the guidelines of Week One on either the fifth, sixth, or seventh day, depending on how many days you committed to fasting during Week Three. The greater the number of days you chose to fast, the more time you should allow to convert to the vegan guidelines from Week One. Most importantly, listen to what your body truly needs rather then automatically following a habit.

EVERY DAY

Throughout the week, use the tools and activities that support your reintegration. For example, refer back to the *ra'yoKa* and *Yoga for Beauty* Poses of the Day (or other new activities) you most enjoyed, choosing one each day. Contemplate the actions you can take to align with your future vision. Read the informational pages that most interest you. And take some time to journal about your experience (at the end of this chapter, you will find the Week Four Reflections section for inspiration).

CUSTOMIZING YOUR REINTEGRATION

FOR THE BEGINNER

Do your best to follow the rules of food combining contained in this chapter, especially as they concern the mixing of starches and proteins. If you choose to consume animal products, then buy free-range, grass-fed, or vegetarian-fed organic animal products (where the animals were consciously raised, not fed their family) and consider treating them as a side dish rather than the focal point of your meal. Also, you could experiment with eating meat only once a week. Or you can continue to incorporate vegan days or at least "meatless Mondays."

FOR THE INTERMEDIATE

With live foods as your bridge back to a vegan diet, focus on a mostly vegan diet until you do your next cleanse. A nonvegan indulgence could be a small amount of raw, unpasteurized dairy, keeping in mind that sheep and goat dairy products are more symbiotic with the human digestive system than dairy products from cows and are usually raised in a more natural environment. If you eat meat on the rare occasion, consider that this animal gave its life for you. Know where it came from, give thanks, and use it as medicine.

FOR THE ADVANCED

Continue with a high percentage of live and blended foods even after the conclusion of the twenty-one-day cleanse; make your transition to integrating live whole foods with cooked foods more gradual. As you reintroduce cooked foods, choose foods that could be eaten live. In addition to vegetables, this includes cooked grains that could be eaten sprouted or soaked (as with sprouted quinoa, wild rice, and buckwheat). Get to know and love the science of your body. Take supplements like vitamin B12, chromium, or deer antler as sources for some of the *jing* (the vital essence I referred to in the previous chapter) that you may have been seeking if you craved or ate animal products. Rather than living to eat, see all of the food you eat as having the purpose of helping you live. Make your mind and body a walking temple and your life a masterpiece.

FOOD COMBINING FOR OPTIMAL DIGESTION

The intention of conscious food combining is to consume foods that mix well in the stomach in order to avoid causing unnecessary stress on the digestive system. This practice respects the natural limits of the body's enzyme stores and the conditions required for the assimilation of nutrients. It is also based on understanding how the body needs to break down different foods in relation to the transit times they typically take to pass through the stomach. Like tending a well-oiled machine, this practice maximizes the body's utilization of the nourishing and cleansing properties of the foods you consume, promoting more efficient digestion, metabolism, absorption, and excretion while reducing toxicity produced in the process.

Although it may not be the most glamorous comparison, this is similar to increasing the gas mileage of our car. When we align with our body's natural requirements for digestion, we free up energy reserves, which can then be directed toward metabolizing, building, and repair. As with a cleanse, where the objective is to detoxify accumulated wastes and residues of years past, proper food combining can unburden the intestines and essentially help our digestion "catch up" with the here and now.

The following keys to food combining are guidelines to consider incorporating into your life. What works best varies from person to person depending on unique sensitivities. Knowing the basic interactions, however, can assist you in having digestive harmony more often than not. Through experimentation and experience, you will discover what works best for your body.

KEYS TO FOOD COMBINING

DRINK LIQUIDS ALONE

Water and other liquids, when consumed with a meal, dilute the digestive enzymes required to digest food. It is recommended that you hydrate between meals, waiting at least a half hour after each meal.

EAT FRUITS ALONE

Fruits are high in sugar and water. They pass through the stomach quickly (in around thirty minutes) if poorly combined. Because they digest so quickly, they should be eaten alone or first, because if, for instance, they are eaten after potatoes or meat (these are already complex to digest), they get stuck in the system, creating gas and bloating as they ferment. When they are eaten alone, especially for breakfast, they support the cleansing process, but when they are eaten for dessert, especially after a heavy, poorly combined meal, they do the opposite. An exception could be adding some fruit to a green salad, as long as you're eating it all on an empty stomach.

CONSUME ANIMAL PROTEINS AND STARCHES SEPARATELY

Certain amino protein chains do well together, such as legumes and grains. However, animal muscle requires a more acidic pH than our bodies have and it is hard to break down, whereas starch requires a more alkaline pH to be broken down in the stomach. Our body calculates each thing as a different category to assimilate, and eating them together is incredibly overwhelming and confusing for our system. Whatever is not used in the digestive system gets stored (perhaps along our lengthy colon), and excess toxins are stored somewhere in the tissue. Consuming these two substances together is like the volatile combo of baking soda and vinegar, and can contribute to intestinal upsets like acid reflux, heartburn, fermentation, and decay of the vital organs. Both combine well with vegetables (proteins are best paired with nonstarchy types) and fermented foods (raw breads, seed cheeses, sprouts, kefir, and sauerkraut). A typical protein and starch meal is steak and potatoes. While it may be a classic meal, as you can see, it is not the ideal combination for digestion.

Your answer to these age-old comfort foods, if you need to eat them, is to eat them separately. If you're eating fish, eat it with vegetables. Eat lamb with salad, eggs with avocados and tomatoes and sprouts, cheese with olives, and bread (gluten free of course) with coconut oil and jam.

ADD FERMENTED FOODS

Rich in enzymes and intestinally friendly flora, these foods aid in digestion and rejuvenation by breaking down waste in the large intestine and helping produce vitamin B12. Think sauerkraut, coconut kefir or yogurt, miso, or kim chee. Soy is best eaten fermented (as miso, natto, and tempeh), as it is the most difficult bean to digest.

A note about food allergies: If you still experience food allergies or sensitivities, take a shot at the "mono diet" regimen for a period of time. As the name implies, with the mono diet you eat only one type of food per meal, which could be several oranges at one sitting, one bowl of black rice at the next, then only kale, only sunflower seeds at the next, and so on. This discipline may seem boring, but when toxicity symptoms pop up, it is often a cue that you need some well-deserved immune system rest, and you will really get a complete understanding of your body's reaction to each food. Remember to keep a journal.

Food Combining: *As a Tool for Personal Growth*

Food combining can have an incredibly therapeutic effect in its ability to deepen our sense of self (mind and body). Eating more intuitively and alleviating old physical and emotional baggage encourage us to live more freely in the present.

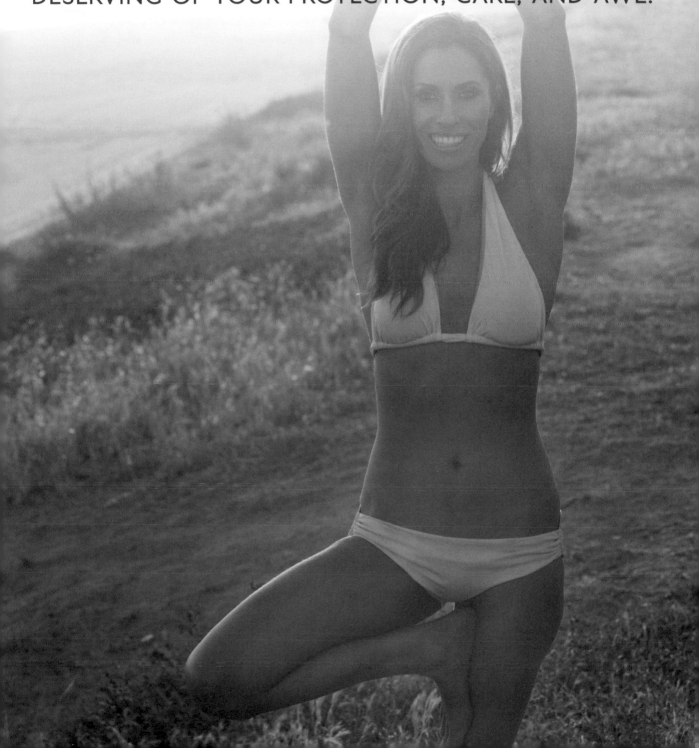

YOUR BODY IS A TEMPLE OF LIGHT,
DESERVING OF YOUR PROTECTION, CARE, AND AWE.

REALIGNING: RETOXING, AND MOVING FORWARD

In our fast-moving world, it's good to remember how much you can gain by taking some things slow and easy, like the steps you choose to take toward optimal health. Just as you would be patient with a toddler who is newly learning to walk, you can also bring patience and kindness to yourself as you continue to take steps toward new ways of eating and living. If you happen to enjoy eating meat and cheese or drinking a glass of wine from time to time, you can still claim your superstar glow! As I have said, being a flexitarian can be a deeply healing path to follow—where our indulgences are warmly met with ever-increasing awareness about what we are eating and its impact on the planet and ourselves. Being a flexitarian doesn't mean that I eat whatever I want, whenever I want. Instead, it means that I do my best to stay on a consistent path that works well for my body. While for me this involves lots of live foods and healthily cooked vegan foods, I'm flexible along the path. Sometimes my focus is on cleansing and lightening up, while at other times it's on building and strengthening. My tastes and needs shift accordingly to what my being and body truly need. In my experience, rigidity of the mind and judgment of self and others can be even more toxic than external pollutants, so I make it a priority to keep a healthy perspective, practice compassion, and allow us all to find what works for each of us.

Remember the rocks in the river we visited at the beginning of this journey together, when the mud had been carried away by the river water and we could then see more clearly the bright shimmering colors of gold, turquoise, and amber? In truth, they were there already, just temporarily covered in mud. I feel confident that if you did this program at even 80 percent of your capacity, you and the people who know you (even helpers at the grocery store and farmers market) are starting to notice that spark about you. People might have asked what you use on your skin or what's different about you. They might notice that you've lost weight. Although we must not get too attached to those compliments, I want you to take a moment to sit with your hard work and deep internal transformation so that you can really experience your own superstar glow. Michelangelo said of his perfect statue of David that the sculpture already existed within the marble stone; he simply removed the excess.

So the choice is yours ... Do you want to continue to shine bright and be a beacon of light for your friends, family, and anyone else you can help and inspire? Or will you cave in to the ego's attempts to sabotage your great work and send you hiding under more stuff as quickly as possible? I have taken both paths at different times and understand their respective joys and perils. So I invite you to see your body as a temple of light, deserving of your protection, care, and awe.

The following ten steps are simple yet highly effective ways to keep moving in the direction of great health—tomorrow, next week, next month, and for years to come.

1. If you are going to eat meat, be mindful of where it's coming from. Choose only free-range, grass-fed (for beef), organic products. Inquire into the practices of the company whose meat you're buying, making sure the animals are not abused, diseased, and injected with hormones and antibiotics (remember: we are what we eat). If you don't need to eat meat, or you're on the fence anyway, try eating a flesh-free diet for another three weeks. If it works for you, keep it up.

2. If you eat dairy, choose unpasteurized, organic products that contain the positive elements of colostrum and fat. Remember that many people are lactose intolerant; symptoms often include excess mucus, recurring ear and/or sinus infections, weight gain, and foul breath. Kids seems to be prone to ear infections due to mucus-forming animal products. Without their parents seeing or understanding the possible connection, they often undergo a series of antibiotics by age ten. Think of yourself as a big kid and honor your body the way you would a child in your care. With so many milk alternatives, consider the fact that even cows switch to grass at three months.

3. If you drink alcohol, choose only organic sources. Red wine (which can be raw) is known for its anti-oxidants—but also sulfites if it's not organic. Or buy the best quality 100 percent agave tequila you can find. In some cultures, this is known as medicine, and if you just sip and absorb with moderation, you will not experience the hangovers that sulfites, chemicals, and excess alcohol produce. Remember in everything, quality over quantity.

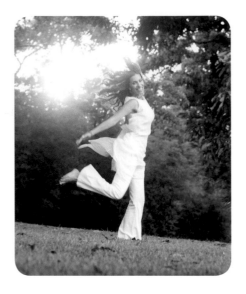

4. If you smoke marijuana for medical purposes, be aware that the hydroponic chemicals and substances used to grow it can be another source of carcinogens, so only choose organic, outdoor-grown sources. And rather than smoke it, use a vaporizer, a machine that uses water vapors instead of smoke and keeps the herb from becoming black. Please remember that by definition the word "medicine" is for treatment, not for a crutch. Anyone who says this substance is not addictive needs to look again. One step away from marijuana would be to vaporize herbs like lavender and sage, and the next would be to drink tonics or take supplements like, for instance, holy basil capsules.

5. If you smoke cigarettes, realize that while the smoke itself is harmful, the 154 chemicals in most cigarettes are even worse. One option is to switch to unadulterated, organic cigarettes or an herbal alternative right away. Cut the amount you smoke in half, get more oxygen, and eventually let the smoking fall away. When you feel like you need a cigarette, do some stretching, jumping jacks, or deep breathing first. You could also try replacing smoking your next cigarette with chewing on a cinnamon stick.

6. If you drink coffee, find an organic, deacidified option. Use nondairy milk sources (like coconut milk creamer) and nonwhite sugars. Simply switch to organic yerba maté or green tea (for me this change was a life saver). Also, notice how the more live, vegan foods you eat, the less you need the stimulant of caffeine to get you up in the morning. Consider using your coffee only for enemas.

7. Chemical sweeteners are considered very toxic, so choose raw sugar, raw honey, agave, coconut sugar, maple syrup, brown rice syrup, dates, figs, raisins, or stevia.

8. If you eat fried food, opt for baked or dehydrated instead. Fried oils tend to be recycled, rancid, and full of toxins that can build up a residue of free radicals in the body, wreaking havoc on organs such as the liver and the skin. On a rare occasion, for a special junk food, try frying sweet potato fries (or other must-haves) in hot coconut oil. Coconut oil can tolerate a higher heat than vegetable oils, which are usually rancid and, quite honestly, toxic.

9. If you eat bread, choose gluten-free options as much as possible and especially those made of rice flour or millet. Spelt is also an option, however, *it does contain gluten*. Although they are related, spelt isn't the same as modern hybridized wheat and is more easily tolerated by people who have a mild sensitivity to wheat. *Note: Spelt is generally not suitable for those with celiac disease.*

10. When choosing grains, the best and most mineral-filled are the darker ones. From black or wild rice to black or red quinoa, colors indicate more phytonutrients.

TAKING IT FURTHER

When you feel ready to pick up the pace and take further steps toward optimal health, the following ideas offer the next level of adjustments you could make.

1. Consider your cravings. <u>We often crave what we are most allergic to.</u>

2. If you do decide that you are eating meat, choose organic, grass-fed meat. Try not eating meat for the next week. If you eat organic, unpasteurized dairy products, try switching to rice or nut alternatives such as almond milk, cashew cheese, or coconut yogurt. If you need to have some dairy, at least make sure that your sources are whole fat (perhaps what you're really craving) and combine with something live and enzyme rich for digestion. Consider drinking a class of lemon juice with your dairy meals.

3. If you drink organic wine and it seems habitual, give yourself a break from it for a few days or weeks, and depending on your habit, designate certain days of the week alcohol free.

4. If you vaporize or still smoke marijuana for medical purposes, try not to do it for a few days, weeks, or longer depending on your current use. You could even seek out alternatives with a naturopath, healer, or shaman, with whom the habit can be met with intention and spiritual awareness.

A special note regarding sacred medicinal plants: Power plants are medicines in which the spirit of the plant is protected and only used in a special ceremony with very clear intentions. Natives of the Amazon know about the benefits and healing properties that come from ingesting these sacred serums of truth while under proper guidance, such as during a vision quest. Interestingly, some addicts have found the root of their suffering and disease by using healing plants such as Ayahuasca and Iboga. One can heal the root of the spiritual misalignment and allow that healing to have an effect on the emotional and physical realms as well. This can take work, but there are skilled guides and even churches that honor this art. I have personally seen many incurable diseases altered through these medicines.

5. If you smoke organic cigarettes, now try herbal cigarettes. And remember those cinnamon sticks to relieve the hand and oral fixation you may be missing.

6. If you drink strong French-pressed yerba maté, switch to tea bags and green tea. Take your morning ritual to the next level by starting your day with eight to sixteen ounces of warm water, a capful of apple cider vinegar, fresh-squeezed lemon, and a touch of raw honey. Add a pinch of cayenne or cinnamon for that extra kick.

7. If you eat lots of dates and honey, stick to organic, 100 percent *really* raw honey and slowly begin to eliminate the dependency on sweeteners. Eat fruits by themselves or in the morning. Sugar and sweet treats don't digest well on a full stomach.

8. If you are still eating white rice, pasta, and refined flours, switch to brown rice and gluten-free products. Raw kelp noodles by Sea Tangle are excellent. If you are already gluten free, trying moving to "live" grains: grains that can be sprouted, such as quinoa, wild rice, and buckwheat. Take it to an even higher level and make a raw bagel with sprouted buckwheat dough and raw strawberry cream cheese made with raw almonds.

9. If you usually grocery shop at large commercial stores, like Costco or Wal-Mart, try supporting locally owned stores like your local co-op and farmers markets for locally grown, organic produce that just came out of the ground or off the tree. The other day, I was talking with a guy who grew the majority of carrots in California. When I asked him about the difference between organic and commercial carrots, he said that he would only eat organic—that the commercial crops get rotated every five years as opposed to three years for organic, and as a result, organic crops contain greater amounts of vitamins and minerals.

10. If you always drive your car to work, try carpooling just once a week, taking the bus, or riding your bike. Make it an adventure!

11. If you watch a lot of TV, try reading a good book that is inspiring and spiritually uplifting. Books are oftentimes the catalysts we need to take that next big life-transforming step. My top three right now are *The Alchemist* (Paulo Coelho), *The Four Agreements* (Miguel Ángel Ruiz), and *Eat, Pray, Love* (Elizabeth Gilbert). Each of these books is very easily digested and yet life changing. You could also go to a movie and enjoy being out in the world.

12. If you are bored or stuck in a rut, try giving more. One of the most inspiring things you can do is to take time one day a week (or even one day a month) to serve an organization you believe in—an inner-city program, school, or other nonprofit. Helping and serving others is the fastest way to help yourself.

A Few Words on Addiction: *What is in the way IS the way*

In chapter 4, I described the teacher training in which I incorporated an adapted version of the twenty-one-day cleanse. While the outcome was spectacular, with students having amazing breakthroughs in their bodies and hearts, there were a few challenging moments on the way to those breakthroughs. One student was plagued for days with strong cravings for cooked food, assuring us that she might not make it without a chicken and cheese burrito. She was also extremely moody, with a lot of anger coming to the surface. We eventually discovered, near the end of the course, that in addition to going through a divorce and recovering from a broken arm, she had some pretty big shadows to face. It turned out that she was also taking various pharmaceutical drugs to ease her emotional and physical pain and had become quite addicted to them. It was a very hard time for her, but she stuck with the process of the training, and she let the power of living foods, yoga, and being surrounded by a loving community of people help her heal. She began to breathe a little more deeply than before, including during those moments when pain, anger, and fear arose. Two months after the training, she decided to go into rehab to address her addiction to the pills head on. She also had a pretty amazing journey in South America with a Peruvian shaman around that time, and perhaps that gave her the tools and the strength necessary to take on rehabilitation.

As the saying goes, pain is inevitable but suffering is not. This brave woman did what we all can do—walk diligently into our blockages, and with breath and love, begin to unravel from the constriction that fear spins and open to our true potential. The power of eating light-filled foods and taking simple steps each day to care for our well-being makes what seemed impossible, possible. It strengthens us to courageously and compassionately face our limitations in order to let them go. It shows us that we are the treasures we are seeking. Through opening up the hidden pockets of our past and addressing our present blockages, we discover how to be free of them.

SUPER TONIC SMOOTHIE

Making a Super Tonic Smoothie can be nutritious and revitalizing.

INGREDIENTS
- 1 cup of organic yogurt (preferably nondairy)
- ½ ripe banana
- ½ teaspoon ginseng powder
- 1 tablespoon raw almond butter
- 1 tablespoon nutritional yeast
- 1 tablespoon maca
- 1 tablespoon tocotrienols

DIRECTIONS
Blend and enjoy!

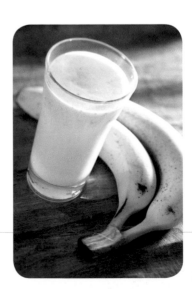

Secrets keep us sick

Major life changes, chronic stress and anxiety, genetics, cultural influences, nutritional deficiencies, allergies, and neurotransmitter imbalances are some of the factors that can be found at the root of an addiction. The longing for deep spiritual connection—when we don't acknowledge and nourish it—can also turn into the cravings of addiction. Disease begins with the ego and manifests spiritually, emotionally, and then physically. Addiction can also bring on psychological and emotional problems, or it can be the result of them. Whatever the case may be, the healing lies in making peace and shining the light that turns lies into truth and secrets into transparency.

Without a doubt, addiction is an intricate dynamic within our human construct. Studies show that there is a correlation between every addiction and blood sugar problems, as well as other nutritional deficiencies. If you have ever been to a support group for people dealing with an addiction, you may have noticed that coffee, cookies, and cigarette breaks are often part of the scene. Almost everyone has been touched by addiction to one degree or another. Whether you can empathize with having an addiction to ice cream, coffee, or something more serious, the following suggestions are offered as ways to address cravings at the physiological level and begin to find the doorway to total freedom.

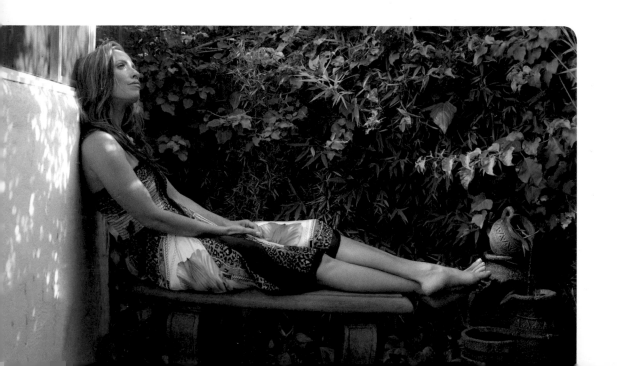

- Eat small, frequent meals, and get more alkaline by consuming lots of fresh fruits and vegetables. Use foods that help the liver clean itself, such as apples, artichokes, beets, burdock root, carrots, celery, daikon radish, green leafy vegetables, persimmons, and flaxseed oil. These foods also help clear excess heat from the body. Sea vegetables help nourish the thyroid gland and endocrine system. Drink the juice of half a lemon in water several times daily. Cleanse, nurture, and rebuild.

- Drink Super Tonic Smoothies (see page 336).

- Superfoods like blue-green algae, spirulina, and chlorella can also be highly nutritive, detoxifying, and rebuilding for those who are giving up an addiction of any sort.

- When giving up an addiction, nurture yourself with high-quality vitamin-mineral supplements. Vitamin C is detoxifying and can reduce cravings. Calcium and magnesium in combination are especially helpful in soothing the nervous system and promoting calmness. B Complex helps diminish withdrawal symptoms and aids liver regeneration. A supplement of GTF (glucose tolerance factor) chromium helps regulate blood sugar levels and metabolize carbohydrates.

- Many contending with addictions are poor oxygen metabolizers and see significant improvements by practicing deep breathing and getting exercise, both of which increase the amount of oxygen available to every cell in the body. The shift can start right now: take a nice deep breath in through your nose … and release it gently through your mouth.

- Consider replacing bad addictions with healthier ones. It might just be a stepping stone, but at least it's going in the right direction. Yoga classes, gym trainings, hypnotherapy, art, acting, rollerskating, swimming, charity work, meditating, cleaning, reading, knitting, support groups, and continuing education could all take one's mind off the addiction to self-abuse and instead create new pathways of positive possibility. Addictions develop as a way to fill a void, so consider that connection is what we are actually looking for.

• Find ways to be good to yourself and give to yourself. Good nutrition, exercise, massage, aromatherapy baths, a foot rub, biofeedback, hypnosis, meditation, and prayer may all be healing on deep levels. Another way to give to yourself is to be in touch with people you love, especially those you may have been out of touch with for some time. While you're relaxing in a fragrant, hot bath, perhaps you could call your grandma or an old friend.

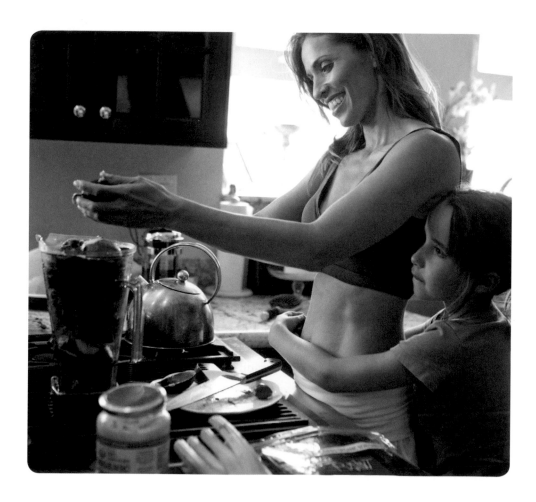

The wisdom of the 12-Step tradition emphasizes taking it "one day at a time." I think the power of this idea can't be overestimated. I know that for myself, I eat living foods and practice yoga every day in order to let go of who I've become and *be* who I really am.

SENDING YOU ON YOUR WAY

When it comes to holding on to old habits and wrestling with addictions, as I shared in the introduction, I get it … I deeply empathize. I know these patterns—both the pain they cause and the fleeting comfort they provide. And there are two questions that I now ask myself when I'm deciding between the life-enhancing thing and the familiar thing, repeating them to myself like a mantra: What do I *love* MORE? What do I *want* MORE? As I continue to delve deeper and deeper into my healing foods lifestyle, the answers for me are unequivocal: What I want more is to be more clear and more aligned and able to give more; to live passionately and embody my destiny. What I want more is to be free. And I choose to focus on these inner truths more than my cravings.

My goal is to awaken, and it's called "spiritual work" for a reason: I must continue to show up for it every day. I'm going to keep practicing the virtues through my food and lifestyle choices, the way I spend my days, and the love and support I extend to those around me. While all of the "sins" are a part of us too, we don't have to choose them. We already know that choosing them leads to suffering and a body that is exhausted and depleted. I want to be my healthy self. I love to be able to run up a flight of stairs. I love to be able to do headstands and handstands. I love having the energy to swim, run, and jump with my daughter. I love eating tons of food—delicious versions of a wide variety of dishes—and appreciating the surplus energy it gives me. A lot of us give in to the lie: the lie about the toll that aging must take. I see people tolerating unnecessary signs of aging, from puffy eyes to chronic disease. But there is another path, and I'm taking it. I choose to be free of the identification of who I'm supposed to be at a certain age. I'm always in a process of metamorphosis. There is a gift I give to myself that consists of five simple words that summarize both a decision about how I live my life and a knowing deep in my soul: I am ageless and eternal.

This gift is for you too. It's your gift. It's right before your eyes. There is a whole world of sensory gifts to enjoy—beautiful things to taste, touch, and feel. So, like pulling on the ribbons of a beautiful package with your name on it, open up the "present" that is the bounty of your life and enjoy it with all of your senses.

Adapting elements of this cleanse to your daily life—and returning to it seasonally—can change your whole life. You can get younger as you get older. Your cells can stop fighting with each other and find harmony. There is a pervasive belief in our world that "healthy" doesn't taste good or that a healthy lifestyle is a restrictive one. But you can change the way you perceive health one bite at a time, literally. You can step outside the paradigm that has people spending a fortune on healthcare and feeling devastated when they don't feel much better —or even find themselves sicker. You can be free to totally recreate yourself.

MY PRAYER IS THAT YOU, AND EVERY PERSON YOU LOVE, KNOW THAT THIS IS POSSIBLE AND SEIZE THE OPPORTUNITY TO MAKE IT SO.

REFLECTIONS
discovering yourself anew

As you did during the three weeks of the cleanse, continue your journey of self-reflection and getting to know yourself in new ways through journaling. The following questions may serve to help you get the pen flowing across the page.

1. What are the biggest changes you have experienced over the past three to four weeks? How have your body, mind, and spirit benefited through this process?

2. What is your plan and how do you intend to stick to it? Lay it all out for yourself.

3. What new virtues, exercises, foods, actions, thoughts, or games did you engage with that you feel move you toward your goals? Do you have more goals? What game will you play with yourself so that you may realize them? Accomplish them?

4. How has your relationship with movement and exercise changed?

5. How has this journey affected the way you perceive your life? Is your sense of purpose stronger? Is your passion for life burning brighter?

6. Has doing the cleanse awakened any new interests? Are there new things you want to learn, places you want to go, or people you would like to meet?

7. Do you have any fears coming up about how to bring your healthy self into the next chapter of your life? Remember that giving voice to your fears can help them to dissipate!

8. Having unleashed more energy during this month, is there a particular new goal that you've set for yourself? What comes next for the SUPERSTAR YOU?

RAINBEAU'S RECIPE ROUNDUP

Welcome to my favorite vegan and raw recipes! In addition to the instructions for each Recipe of the Day (highlighted in the daily schedules for the twenty-one cleanse days), you will find step-by-step directions for each of the glow-enhancing entrées, soups, salads, snacks, sides, toppings, breakfast options, desserts, shakes, smoothies, juices, and tonics that are suggested throughout the cleanse. I have also included bonus recipes that you will only find here in the Roundup, so I encourage you to peruse every page of this mouthwatering section so you don't miss a thing! Each recipe is selected with your greatest health and pleasure in mind—a sumptuous collection to fuel the life you love.

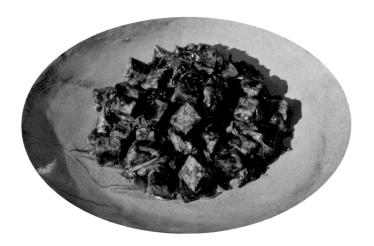

ENTRÉES

BBQ TEMPEH AND GREENS SAUTÉ

INGREDIENTS

- 1 package of tempeh, sliced to make short strips ¼ inch thick
- 1 cup vegan BBQ sauce (recipe below or buy ready-made)
- 2 teaspoons olive oil (extra virgin, cold pressed)
- ¼ cup pure water
- 3 cups collard greens and/or Swiss chard
- 3 cups kale
- 1 onion, diced
- 1 clove garlic, minced
- ½ lemon, juiced
- 3 tablespoons nama shoyu, tamari, or Bragg Liquid Aminos
- 1 tablespoon apple cider vinegar
- Pinch of Celtic sea salt
- Pinch of black pepper (ground peppercorns if possible)

INGREDIENTS—VEGAN BBQ SAUCE

- 1 cup macadamia nuts, cashews, or almonds (soaked overnight)
- 1 cup pure water
- 1 tablespoon lemon juice
- 3 tablespoons mesquite powder
- 2 to 3 cloves garlic
- 2 tomatoes
- ⅛ cup apple cider vinegar
- ¼ cup raw honey, coconut sugar, agave, or maple syrup
- Pinch of Celtic sea salt
- Pinch of black pepper (ground peppercorns)
- Pinch of ground cayenne pepper
- Pinch of ground allspice

Blend together until smooth

DIRECTIONS

1. Combine tempeh and BBQ sauce in a bowl, stirring gently to coat all sides of tempeh slices, and let marinate for 5 minutes.
2. Massage kale and collard greens with oil, salt, and lemon juice.
3. Sauté onions and garlic in a frying pan with oil, then add tempeh and grill until each side is golden brown (about 4 to 5 minutes per side). Then add greens mixture, cooking until leaves are wilted.
4. Season with tamari, apple cider vinegar, and salt and pepper as desired.
5. Serve BBQ tempeh laid over the bed of greens and garnish with a drizzle of BBQ sauce and sautéed onions.

RECIPE OF THE DAY: **BLACK BEAN VEGAN BURGER PATTIES**

This vegan version of the ever-popular burger is earthy, grounding, and delectable!

INGREDIENTS (MAKES 6 BURGERS)

- 2 cups black beans (soaked overnight for 8 hours, rinsed and drained)
- 2 carrots, grated
- ½ cup dry rolled oats (*note: oats are not gluten free*)
- 1 tablespoon olive oil
- Add ½ teaspoon each of your preferred spices: cinnamon, cumin, coriander, chili powder, onion powder, black pepper and cayenne pepper (¼ teaspoon of the peppers)
- 1 teaspoon Celtic sea salt

DIRECTIONS

1. Preheat oven to 300° F.
2. Grate the carrots, then add oats, ¾ cup of the beans, all spices, and the olive oil—mixing all together in the food processor.
3. Spoon mixture into a mixing bowl and then fold in the rest of the whole, reserved beans. Wet your hands and form into 6 medium sized patties.
4. Bake at 300° F for 40 minutes, turning once in the middle.
5. If preferred, prebake for 30 minutes and cook for final heat on the grill until lightly browned.
6. Add to sprouted wheat buns and enjoy. Perfect for vegan cookouts in the spring. Serve with a side or fresh herb salad, which makes an excellent addition to anything you're eating (there is a salad I eat so often that I've given it my own name—Rainbeau's Favorite Herb Salad on page 320).

RECIPE OF THE DAY: **CHEESY VEGETABLE MEDLEY**

This nutritiously filling dish is the perfect marriage of crunchy and creamy.

Note: Although this dish is better in the dehydrator, if you don't have one, there are options. You can put it in a window in the hot sun or outside in the sun (covered with a screen to protect from bugs). A friend of mine used a thermometer to check the heat of her stove while warmed only from the pilot light, and it was 115° F exactly—where there is a will, there is a way. Regarding dehydrators, you can buy them inexpensively nowadays, so consider making the investment for your health ... and for the pleasure of your taste buds.

INGREDIENTS—VEGETABLE MEDLEY

- 1 baby bok choy
- ½ cauliflower
- 2 carrots
- 2 zucchini
- 1 cup olive oil
- Celtic sea salt

INGREDIENTS—NUT CHEESE

- 1 cup macadamia or other raw nut
- 1 tablespoon lemon juice
- 2 garlic cloves
- 2 tablespoons olive oil
- Coriander to taste
- Curry to taste
- Chili pepper to taste

(Recipe continued on next page)

(Continued from previous page)

DIRECTIONS

1. Cut up the vegetables and marinate in olive oil and salt.
2. While the vegetables are marinating, blend the ingredients for nut cheese
3. Cover the vegetables with the nut cheese and mix well.
4. Dehydrate the mixture until the vegetables are softened (about 4 hours).

RECIPE OF THE DAY: COCONUT CURRY WITH BOK CHOY

The blending of coconut and curry could be considered ambrosia of the gods … and goddesses.

INGREDIENTS

- ½ a medium onion
- 1 bunch bok choy
- 1 clove garlic
- 8 ounces tempeh
- ¾ cup coconut milk
- 2 tablespoons coconut oil
- 1 cup diced heirloom tomatoes
- ½ teaspoon curry powder
- 1 teaspoon garam masala
- 1 teaspoon grated ginger (optional)
- Pinch of Celtic sea salt to taste

DIRECTIONS

1. Sauté tempeh in coconut oil in skillet until browned on all sides.
2. Dice the onion and the crunchy stalks of the bok choy and add to the skillet to cook until soft.
3. Chop and set aside the bok choy leaves.
4. Blend the garlic clove, curry, garam masala, ginger, and tomatoes in a blender or food processor until smooth.
5. Once onions and bok choy are soft, add tomato mixture and chopped bok choy leaves to the skillet.
6. When leaves are wilted, add coconut milk; cook until heated through.
7. Season to taste with salt, and serve over brown rice or quinoa—and of course your favorite side salad for the enzymes.

EASY VEGAN QUESADILLAS

INGREDIENTS

- 2 to 4 corn tortillas (sprouted grain if possible)
- ½ cup Daiya cheese or vegan cheese of choice
- 1 avocado
- 2 tablespoons olive oil
- 1 clove of garlic (minced) or garlic powder seasoning

DIRECTIONS

1. Spread cheese between tortillas and place on grill heated to high.
2. Flip after about 3 minutes to cook evenly on each side or until cheese is melted.
3. Serve with sliced avocado, celery sticks, and salsa.

Option: Fill quesadillas with chopped mushrooms, leeks, and/or bok choy sautéed in frying pan with olive oil and garlic.

RECIPE OF THE DAY: **GREEN NOODLES**

A power-packed live food feast for beauty and nutritional replenishment.

INGREDIENTS

- 1 package kelp noodles or 3 zucchini (cut in spirals)
- 1 cup soaked almonds
- 2 cups kale
- 1 heirloom tomato
- ½ cup red bell pepper
- ½ avocado
- 1 tablespoon olive oil
- ½ tablespoon Bragg Liquid Aminos (or nama shoyu or tamari)
- ½ tablespoon lemon juice
- 2 cloves garlic
- Cayenne pepper to taste

DIRECTIONS

1. Add everything except the noodles of choice to the blender and blend.
2. Add the blended dressing on top of the noodles and enjoy!

Option: If you have one, warm in the dehydrator for a couple hours or until warm and soft.

RECIPE OF THE DAY: **GRILLED CHEES-INI SANDWICH**

Enjoy this vegan variation on the classic grilled cheese sandwich.

INGREDIENTS

- ⅓ cup water
- 4 teaspoons nutritional yeast
- 1 tablespoon oat flour—can be a spoon of oats whizzed in the blender (*note: oats and oat flour are not gluten free; omit if gluten sensitive*)
- 1 tablespoon fresh lemon juice
- 1 tablespoon tahini
- 2 teaspoons tomato paste or ketchup
- 1 teaspoon cornstarch
- ½ teaspoon onion granules
- ⅛ teaspoon garlic granules
- ⅛ teaspoon turmeric
- ⅛ teaspoon dry mustard
- ⅛ teaspoon Celtic sea salt
- 4 slices of gluten free bread

DIRECTIONS

1. Place all the ingredients minus the bread in a saucepan and whisk together until the mixture is smooth. Bring to a boil.
2. While stirring constantly, reduce the heat to low. Cook until the cheese sauce is thick and smooth, then remove from heat.
3. Cover one side of each piece of bread with the cheese sauce.
4. Grill the sandwiches in a skillet or toaster oven and serve with some veggies on the side.

For a quick grilled cheese, try just grilling the bread on a griddle or skillet with coconut oil, sprinkle with your preferred type of Daiya cheese, and place one piece of the bread on top of the Daiya. Add whatever else you might like in the sandwich or as a side.

KELP NOODLE STIR-FRY

INGREDIENTS

- 1 package kelp noodles
- 3 cups spinach
- 1 to 2 tomatoes, diced
- 2 onions, thinly sliced
- 1 cup mushrooms, sliced, optional
- 1 cup carrots, julienned
- 2 cloves garlic, minced
- 3 tablespoons sesame or coconut oil
- ½ lemon, juiced
- 2 tablespoons nama shoyu, tamari, or Bragg Liquid Aminos
- Pinch of Celtic sea salt
- 1 teaspoon raw honey, agave, or maple syrup

DIRECTIONS

Marinate noodles, onions, and mushrooms in a mixture of lemon juice, tamari, salt, and oil for 5 to 15 minutes.

Cooked option: In a frying pan over medium heat, sauté together with remaining ingredients for 5 minutes or until noodles are soft.

Raw option: Simply toss together with remaining ingredients and serve.

RECIPE OF THE DAY: **LIVE SPRING ROLLS**

An Asian-influenced meal that is easy to make and bursting with flavor and crunch.

INGREDIENTS—ROLL FILLING

- ½ bunch collard greens
- 2 to 3 carrots, julienned
- ¼ head purple cabbage, shredded
- ¾ cup minced almonds

INGREDIENTS—SAUCE

- ¼ cup onions, mashed (to release flavor)
- 2 tablespoons nama shoyu
- 2 tablespoons sweetener (maple syrup is great in this, and although not live, it's mineral rich)
- 1 teaspoon toasted sesame oil, or chopped almonds as an alternate
- ½ juiced orange

DIRECTIONS

1. Wash the collard green leaves and remove the hard stems.
2. Toss all the chopped vegetables in half the sauce for a more decadent option, or simply keep to the side for dipping.
3. Fill the leaves with the carrots, cabbage, almonds, and anything else you would like to put inside.
4. Roll the leaves into spring roll shapes to contain the filling.
5. Mix the sauce ingredients together in a separate bowl.
6. Dip the rolls in the remainder of the sauce. Enjoy!

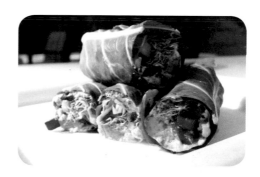

RAW FAJITAS

INGREDIENTS—VEGETABLES

Choose from ...

- Bell peppers
- Tomatoes
- Avocados
- Zucchini or yellow squash marinated in nama shoyu and olive oil
- Jalapeños or chili peppers (according to your spice comfort level)
- Lettuce or cabbage leaves
- Olive oil
- Celtic sea salt
- Cayenne or chili powder
- Live Vegan Sour Cream (page 322)

DIRECTIONS

1. According to your selection of veggies, cut up bell peppers, squash, tomatoes, avocados, and jalapeños.
2. Use lettuce or cabbage leaves as your tortillas.
3. Adorn with a touch of olive oil, a pinch of Celtic sea salt, and a sprinkle of cayenne or chili powder.
4. Complete with a dollop of Vegan Sour Cream, and enjoy!

RAW PIZZA *Recipe contributed by Brigitte Mars*

INGREDIENTS—PIZZA CRUST

- 1½ cups sprouted buckwheat
- ¼ cup extra virgin olive oil
- ⅔ cup zucchini
- 2 cloves garlic (optional)
- 1 tablespoon basil
- 1 teaspoon oregano
- 1 tablespoon rosemary
- 1 teaspoon Celtic sea salt
- ⅔ cup flaxseeds, soaked in 1⅓ cup water for 15 minutes

INGREDIENTS—TOMATO SAUCE

(can also be used with raw pasta; makes 3 cups)

- 4 large tomatoes
- ½ cup sun-dried tomatoes, soaked 2 hours
- 3 tablespoons extra virgin olive oil
- ¼ cup fresh basil
- 2 cloves garlic
- 1 teaspoon anise or fennel seed
- 3 dates, soaked 20 minutes
- 1 teaspoon Celtic sea salt
- Combine all ingredients in a food processor or blender and puree.

DIRECTIONS

1. Combine all pizza crust ingredients except the flaxseeds in a food processor and puree.
2. Empty the contents of the food processor into a bowl and add the flaxseeds. Mix well.
3. Form into 2 large round pizza crusts on solid dehydrator sheets. Dehydrate 7 to 8 hours, or until crispy on one side. Turn, remove the dehydrator sheets, and dry another 7 to 8 hours.
4. Spread the sauce over the crusts. Other sauce options: Herb Pesto (page 322) or Alfredo Sauce (page 321)
5. Finally, add the toppings of your choice. I like to top raw pizza with an almond Nut Cheese (page 323), chopped basil, sun-dried tomatoes, sun-cured olives, tomato slices, avocado slices, oregano, pine nuts, edible flowers, and marinated eggplant or mushrooms. Makes 2 pizzas.

RECIPE OF THE DAY: **RED GRAPE VEGAN TACOS** *Recipe contributed by Aisha*

INGREDIENTS—MAIN SALAD FOR THE TACOS

- ½ large jicama, peeled and thinly sliced (about 1½ cups)
- 1 cup cilantro leaves and stems, finely chopped
- ½ cup red seedless grapes (organic), halved
- ½ avocado, diced
- 1 lime, juiced
- 1 tablespoon olive oil (optional)
- Finely diced jalapeño
- Dash of smoked paprika
- Salt and pepper to taste

INGREDIENTS—TORTILLAS AND CONDIMENTS

- 4 corn or rice tortillas
- 1 cup fresh chopped tomato salsa (chopped tomato, onion, garlic, and cilantro)
- 1 can black beans, drained and warmed on stovetop for a few minutes
- 1 cup guacamole (chopped avocado, tomato, lime juice, cilantro, salt and pepper to taste)
- Vegan sour cream
- Vegan shredded cheese, such as Daiya

DIRECTIONS

1. Combine all main salad ingredients in a large bowl and toss well.
2. Chill for at least a half hour to allow flavors to marinate and mix.
3. Warm tortillas on the stove or in the oven, sprinkling with vegan shredded cheese (cheese optional).
4. Assemble the tacos to your liking and enjoy with friends!

SOBA PASTA WITH TAHINI MISO SAUCE

INGREDIENTS

- 1 package soba noodles (buckwheat or gluten free)
- 2 cups pure water
- 3 tablespoons miso paste (unpasteurized)
- 3 tablespoons tahini butter
- 2 tablespoons coconut or sesame oil
- 1 clove of garlic, minced
- ½ cup sesame seeds
- 2 to 3 tablespoons nama shoyu, tamari, or Bragg Liquid Aminos
- 4 green onions, chopped
- 3 cups broccoli florets
- ½ cup shredded carrots
- 1 cup sliced green beans
- 1 tomato, sliced

DIRECTIONS

1. Preheat oven to 375° F and pour the sesame seeds onto a rimmed baking sheet.
2. Toast the seeds in the oven for 10 to 12 minutes, until they are a rich brown around the edges.
3. Boil water and add soba noodles, cooking for about 5 minutes or until soft. Drain and rinse with cool water and drain again.
4. For your pasta sauce, blend miso, oil, tahini, nama shoyu or other sauce, and water.
5. Sauté soba noodles in frying pan with oil, 1 tablespoon nama shoyu or other sauce, sesame seeds, garlic, broccoli, carrots, and green beans.
6. Pour mixture in a bowl, drizzle with creamy tahini miso sauce, and serve with raw tomato slices.

SPROUTARONI *Recipe contributed by Brigitte Mars*

INGREDIENTS

- 2 cups sunflower sprouts
- 1 cup cashews
- Juice of 1 lemon
- Big pinch of Celtic sea salt
- 1 teaspoon sauerkraut
- ½ cup water
- 2 teaspoons olive oil

DIRECTIONS

1. Blend until smooth, adding water until you have a smooth texture without any lumps.
2. Enjoy!

SUPREME VEGAN BURRITO

INGREDIENTS

- 1 whole avocado
- 1 whole tomato
- 1 bunch of cilantro or basil
- 1 teaspoon cumin
- 1 teaspoon Celtic sea salt
- 1 clove garlic
- 2 tablespoons tofu sour cream
- 1 whole green or red pepper
- Drizzle of nama shoyu or Bragg Liquid Aminos
- 2 sprouted-grain wheat or corn tortillas

DIRECTIONS

1. Slice and dice produce.
2. Warm tortillas in a frying pan, then fill with prepped ingredients. ¡Qué bueno!

THAI NOODLE DELIGHT *Recipe contributed by Brigitte Mars, from her book* Rawsome!

This is a dish with staying-power. If you store the noodles separate from the sauce, it makes for a great lunch or dinner the next day.

INGREDIENTS—NOODLES

- 2 cups white cabbage
- 2 cups red cabbage
- 2 cups noodle like slivers of coconut meat
- ½ cup chopped fresh cilantro
- ½ cup chopped fresh basil

INGREDIENTS—SAUCES

- 1-inch piece of fresh ginger root
- 6 dates, presoaked for 20 minutes
- 2 tablespoons tamarind paste (soaked for 20 minutes in 3 tablespoons water, lemon juice, or lime juice ... lime is my personal favorite); do not drain
- 2 tablespoons nama shoyu
- ½ cup orange juice
- ¼ teaspoon cayenne
- ¼ cup tahini or almond butter
- ¼ cup cashews or almond nuts for garnish

DIRECTIONS

1. Grate the cabbage.
2. To make the base, toss the coconut, cabbage, and herbs in a large bowl.
3. To make the sauce, puree all the sauce ingredients together.
4. To finish, pour the sauce over the coconut and cabbage noodles and garnish with nuts. Yields 4 servings.

RECIPE OF THE DAY: **VEGAN PIZZA**

Because I want you to realize that there are always healthier versions of everything, we're going to kick off the cleanse with a crowd pleaser.

INGREDIENTS – TOPPING CHOICES

· 2 large tomatoes, cut in half and sliced
· 2 garlic cloves, crushed
· Handful of fresh basil leaves
· Daiya cheese, mozzarella (optional)
· Grain sausage substitute (optional)
· 1 container pizza sauce or regular tomato sauce (or even salsa)

For extra "veggie love" try chopped onions, eggplants, zucchini, and peppers.

INGREDIENTS—CRUST

2 wheat-free crusts can be found in most grocery stores; you'll usually want enough for other people and leftovers. Rice crust is great, and cornmeal is yummy too, yet usually contains some wheat.

DIRECTIONS

1. Preheat the oven to 425° F.
2. Take the crusts out of wrappers.
3. Spoon on evenly the pizza or tomato sauce or salsa
4. Place the tomatoes and sprinkle on garlic and basil and cover with Daiya cheese.
5. Use the veggies and experiment with a grain sausage on one or, if you love them, both of the crusts.
6. Place in middle of oven for about 10 minutes—and standby while shredding romaine lettuce to serve on the side.
7. For the extra veggies, grill the chopped onions in coconut oil until clear and then add the rest of the cubed veggies. Let sit and cool until needed before topping pizza.
8. Play it cool as friends beg to join the cleanse.

RECIPE OF THE DAY: **VEGETABLE TEMPEH KEBOBS SKEWER**

This dish is a perfect merging of distinctive flavors and satisfying textures. Enjoy!

INGREDIENTS

· 1 package tempeh
· 8 wooden skewers (soak in water to make skewering easier)
· 4 cubed portobello or shiitake mushrooms
· ½ zucchini (cut in half lengthwise)
· ½ red onion cut into ½-inch chunks
· ½ red pepper, large dice
· ½ yellow pepper, large dice
· 8 cherry tomatoes

INGREDIENTS—MARINADE

· 6 tablespoons wheat-free tamari
· 1 cup apple juice
· ¾ cup orange juice (2 oranges)
· 4 to 8 cloves garlic, minced
· 2 tablespoons Dijon mustard
· 3 tablespoons minced fresh rosemary or 1 tablespoon, dried
· 1 cup liquid coconut oil or olive oil (½ cup for marinade, remaining for vegetables)

DIRECTIONS

1. Cut the tempeh in half.
2. Place the tempeh into a pot with the marinade and simmer for 30 minutes.
3. Cube simmered tempeh into 4 cubes (for a total of 8) after it cools.
4. Add oil to marinade and marinate vegetables for an hour or more.
5. Create kebobs using vegetables and 1 cube of tempeh per skewer.
6. Grill 5 minutes on each side and serve warm or at room temperature.

ZUCCHINI SPAGHETTI WITH MARINARA

INGREDIENTS

- 2 to 3 zucchini (peeled and spiralized)
- 2 to 3 large tomatoes
- 1 date
- 1 tablespoon olive oil
- ½ to 1 cup of water
- ½ teaspoon miso
- ¼ teaspoon red pepper
- 1 teaspoon Celtic sea salt
- 3 to 4 sun-dried tomatoes (soaked)
- 5 sun-dried olives (take out pits and chop)

DIRECTIONS

1. Place everything but the olives in a Vitamix (or other high-speed blender) or food processor. Using a food processor with the "S" blade yields a more chunky sauce, while the Vitamix will make it creamy smooth very quickly.
2. Pulse until you reach desired texture.
3. Peel the zucchinis and use a spiralizer to create long spirals of spaghetti-like noodles.
4. In a bowl, toss the zucchini noodles, sauce, olives, and more oil to taste. Enjoy!

SOUPS

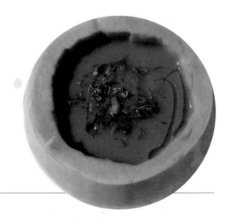

BUTTERNUT SQUASH BISQUE

INGREDIENTS

- 1 butternut squash (peeled and cubed)
- 1 onion (chopped)
- 2 cups pure water or vegetable broth
- ½ cup celery (finely chopped)
- 2 tablespoons coconut or olive oil
- Pinch of Celtic sea salt
- Pinch of black pepper (from ground peppercorns)
- Pinch of ground allspice
- 1 sprig fresh thyme, rosemary, and sage (optional)
- 1 cup coconut milk (or almond, rice, or soy milk)

DIRECTIONS

1. Sauté the onion, celery, thyme, rosemary, and sage in the olive oil with salt and pepper for about 5 minutes or until the herbs are tender.
2. Add the butternut squash and broth to the pan. Simmer the mixture on medium-low heat for 20 minutes, until squash is tender.
3. Pour the mixture into your Vitamix or other blender, add the coconut milk, and puree the soup until completely smooth.
4. Serve garnished with a sprig of sage and flax crackers.

RECIPE OF THE DAY: **CELERY CHOWDER**

With garlic and cayenne adding the heat, this soup recipe is warming and awakening.

INGREDIENTS

· 1 cup macadamia nuts
· 8 stalks celery: 5 to 6 chopped for blending, and 2 to 3, diced
· 2 chopped squash
· 2 cloves garlic
· ½ avocado
· Pinch Celtic sea salt
· Cayenne to taste
· 1 sprig rosemary or to taste
· 1 teaspoon extra virgin olive oil

DIRECTIONS

1. Combine all the ingredients except the diced celery into a blender with enough water to completely cover everything.
2. Blend everything until smooth and creamy. Add water to change the consistency.
3. Stir the diced celery into the soup for extra texture.
4. Add a few slices of avocado on top and drizzle on some olive oil for a final touch.

You can heat this soup on the stove to slightly warm it up if you desire, taking care not to heat it to the point where it would no longer be considered raw.

ENERGY SOUP

INGREDIENTS

· 1 avocado
· 1 carrot
· 1 to 2 tomatoes
· 1 lemon
· 1 bunch of sprouts
· 1 bunch of kale
· Peppers of your choice
· Sliver of papaya
· Cilantro, basil, or any other preferred fresh herbs
· Himalayan or Celtic salt
· Unpasteurized miso
· 1 handful of soaked raw almonds
· 1 small handful of your favorite seaweed

DIRECTIONS

1. In your blender, mix your choice of ingredients at a pulse, taking care not to overblend.
2. Create any version of this you like for real, live energy!

MAGICAL MERMAID SOUP

INGREDIENTS

· 3 cups coconut water or pure water
· 2 tablespoons coconut oil
· ¼ cup dulse or kelp seaweed
· ¼ cup nori, shredded
· ¼ daikon, shredded
· Pinch of Celtic sea salt (optional)
· 1 teaspoon miso (recommended brand: Shaman Shack Herbs Sea Clear, with fermented kelp and chlorella)

DIRECTIONS

1. In blender, combine coconut water, coconut oil, miso, and dulse or kelp. Blend until smooth.
2. Stir in shredded nori and daikon and a pinch of salt and serve.

MEXICALI SOUP

INGREDIENTS

- 2 to 3 celery stalks
- 1 to 2 avocados
- 1 ripe tomato
- Corn from one cob
- 1 tablespoon olive oil
- 1 teaspoon cumin
- 1 dash of cayenne, chili powder and/or paprika
- Celtic sea salt to taste
- Handful of chopped cilantro leaves (optional)
- 2 cups of pure water, slightly warmed

DIRECTIONS

1. Place all these ingredients in the food processor and pulse until blended but still with texture and chunks.
2. Spice to your liking and enjoy!

MEXICAN AVOCADO SOUP

INGREDIENTS

- 1 whole avocado
- 1 whole tomato
- 1 bunch of cilantro or basil
- 1 teaspoon cumin
- 1 teaspoon Celtic sea salt
- 1 cup pure water
- 1 clove of garlic
- Corn kernels from one fresh cob (optional)

DIRECTIONS

Put everything in the food processor and pulse until it combines. Go slowly to ensure that your mixture remains somewhat whole and not overly blended.

MORNING MISO SOUP

INGREDIENTS

- 3 cups pure water
- 3 tablespoons miso paste (unpasteurized)
- 1 tablespoon nutritional yeast
- ½ package of tofu, diced (optional)
- 2 tablespoons olive oil
- 1 clove garlic, minced
- 2 green onions, sliced
- 1 avocado (optional)

DIRECTIONS

1. Boil water. After it has cooled a bit, stir in miso, olive oil, nutritional yeast, and preferred seasonings to make broth. *Special note: never boil miso.*
2. Add tofu chunks, green onions, and smashed avocado as desired.

QUICK RAW TOMATO SOUP

INGREDIENTS

- 2 large red tomatoes
- 1 tablespoon extra virgin olive oil
- 1 clove of garlic
- 1 red pepper
- 1 teaspoon nutritional yeast
- A hit of ponzu (Japanese citrus-based sauce)
- 1 cup pure water
- Chopped basil and Celtic sea salt to taste

DIRECTIONS

1. Place all ingredients in the Vitamix or blender until smooth.
2. Use your creative imagination and garnish the soup as you are so inspired. My personal favorite way to eat this soup is to crumble good seed cheese on top and add a splash of olive oil and cayenne. I especially enjoy the nourishing warmth of this combo when the seasons change.

RAW COOLING GAZPACHO

INGREDIENTS

- 1 whole tomato, chopped
- 1 whole cucumber, chopped (if organic, keep the skin on; it's a beauty food!)
- 2 to 3 tablespoons olive oil
- 1 clove of garlic
- 1 teaspoon Celtic sea salt
- 1 bunch of cilantro or basil
- 1 cup pure water
- Juice of half a lemon

DIRECTIONS

1. Put everything in the food processor and pulse until it combines. Go slowly to ensure that your mixture remains somewhat whole and not overly blended.
2. Option: For a superfood boost, include a scoop of Vitamineral Green from HealthForce Nutritionals.

RECIPE OF THE DAY: RAW PROSPERITY SOUP

This warming and lively soup is nourishing to kidneys, bladder, reproductive system, lungs, and creativity.

INGREDIENTS

- 1 cup chopped carrots
- 1½ cups coconut water (young Thai coconut)
- ½ cup coconut meat (young Thai coconut)
- 1 orange
- ½ cup walnuts or almonds, soaked and rinsed
- 1 teaspoon ginger
- 1 teaspoon cinnamon
- 1 clove garlic (optional)
- 2 tablespoons raw honey, maple syrup, or a few dates (optional)

DIRECTIONS

Blend all of the ingredients until creamy. Before eating, bless your soup with: *I allow abundance and prosperity into my life.*

SALADS

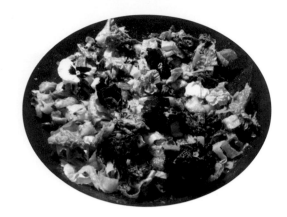

CREAMY AVOCADO KALE SALAD

INGREDIENTS—SALAD

- 1 bunch kale
- ½ lemon
- 1 tomato, diced
- ½ cucumber, diced
- 1 to 2 avocados, ripe
- 1 handful mushrooms, shiitake or maitake (optional)
- ½ cup diced eggplant (optional)
- 2 tablespoons coconut oil (extra virgin, cold pressed)
- 2 tablespoons mama shoyu, tamari, or Bragg Liquid Aminos
- 1 tablespoon nutritional yeast
- Pinch of Celtic sea salt
- Pinch of parsley or cilantro
- Choice of vegan salad dressing or Creamy Dreamy Dressing (recipe to right).

INGREDIENTS—CREAMY DREAMY DRESSING

- 1 cup macadamia nuts, cashews, or almonds, soaked overnight
- 1 to 2 cups pure water
- 1 tablespoon lemon juice
- Pinch of Celtic sea salt
- 1 clove garlic (optional)

Blend together until smooth

DIRECTIONS

1. With clean hands, massage shredded kale with oil, salt, and lemon juice.
2. Marinate mushrooms and/or eggplant with oil and tamari before adding to mixture.
3. Toss salad with remaining ingredients and drizzle with your dressing of choice.

DELIGHTFUL FRUIT SALAD

INGREDIENTS

- ⅓ cup watermelon, cubed
- ⅓ cup raw honeydew melon, cubed
- ⅓ cup cantaloupe, cubed
- 1 to 2 kiwis, cubed
- ¼ cup blueberries (optional)
- ¼ cup goji berries (optional)
- 1 orange, sliced (optional)
- Pinch of Celtic sea salt

DIRECTIONS

Combine fruit medley in a bowl ... and be light!

EASY KALE SALAD

INGREDIENTS

- 1 avocado
- 1 bunch kale
- ½ lemon
- 1 tablespoon olive oil
- Pinch Celtic sea salt

DIRECTIONS

1. Chop the avocado and kale into bite-sized pieces and place in mixing bowl.
2. Drizzle with lemon juice, olive oil, and sea salt, then massage until thoroughly marinated. Bon appétit!

Option: Add tomatoes and your favorite herbs. Toss in some hemp seeds for added protein.

RECIPE OF THE DAY: **KALE & AVOCADO SALAD**

Enjoy the superior nutritional profile of this hearty and flavorful salad.

INGREDIENTS

- ½ bunch kale
- 1 ripe avocado
- ¼ onion, chopped
- ¼ cup shredded purple cabbage
- ¼ cup olive oil
- ½ lemon, juiced
- ½ teaspoon nama shoyu
- 1 tablespoon sweetener of choice (raw honey, agave, etc.)
- Sesame seeds for garnish

DIRECTIONS

1. Break the kale into bite-sized pieces, chop the avocado into small pieces.
2. Combine the kale, avocado, onions, and purple cabbage into one bowl.
3. Mix the olive oil, lemon juice, nama shoyu, and sweetener together in a separate bowl to create a dressing/marinade for the salad.
4. Use clean hands to massage the marinade into the kale and all the other veggies until soft.
5. Let the salad marinate for about an hour.

Option: If you have leftovers, you can dehydrate and make delicious veggie chips by simply spreading the mixture onto a dehydrator tray.

QUEEN (QUINOA) AND KING (KALE) SALAD

INGREDIENTS

- 3 cups of pure water
- 1 cup quinoa, soaked overnight
- 2 cups kale
- 2 tablespoons olive oil (extra virgin, cold pressed)
- Pinch of Celtic sea salt
- ½ lemon
- 1 tomato, diced
- ⅓ cup olives, sliced
- Pinch of dill, rosemary, mint, and fennel to taste

DIRECTIONS

1. Boil water, stir in quinoa, and let simmer until soft. Then rinse with cool water.
2. With clean hands, massage shredded kale with olive oil, salt, and lemon juice.
3. Toss prepared kale with remaining herbs, tomato, olives, and quinoa. Serve and enjoy.

RECIPE OF THE DAY: **RAINBEAU'S FAVORITE HERB SALAD**

So simple, delicious, aromatic, and healing … I make this salad all the time now and eat it as a main dish, although it also makes a beautiful garnish for any meal.

INGREDIENTS

- · 1 bunch of fresh parsley
- · 1 bunch of fresh mint
- · 1 bunch of fresh basil
- · 1 bunch of cilantro (optional)
- · 1 bunch of fresh dill
- · 1 lemon
- · ¼ cup extra virgin olive oil, or to taste
- · Celtic sea salt to taste

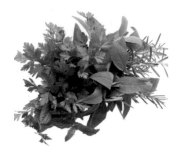

DIRECTIONS

1. De-stem all these amazing plants and then start chopping. *Note: If you can, use a ceramic knife, as it keeps these herbs from turning brown.*
2. Toss into a bowl together and add in a liberal amount of olive oil, lemon, and Celtic sea salt. Herbs tend to absorb quickly, so depending on the amount of fresh herbs you're using, modify these flavor-enhancing and preserving condiments.

Goodness … even as I write I wish I had some ready to eat. This lively salad makes you feel clean and refreshed from the inside out.

WILD RICE HARMONY

INGREDIENTS

- · 3 cups wild rice, soaked for 8 hours or overnight
- · 1 cup hearts of palm, chopped in chunks
- · 1 cup artichoke hearts, chopped in chunks
- · 3 tablespoons or liberal amount olive oil or truffle oil
- · 1 teaspoon Celtic sea salt
- · 1 tablespoon nama shoyu, tamari, or Bragg Liquid Aminos

DIRECTIONS

1. Soak wild rice for approximately 8 hours, rinse, and add to mixing bowl.
2. Chop hearts of palm and artichoke hearts into chunks and add to rice.
3. Pour at least 3 tablespoons olive oil, sea salt, and nama shoyu or other sauce over mixture.
4. Use spoons or tongs to toss mixture until all rice and hearts are thoroughly dressed. Serve and enjoy!

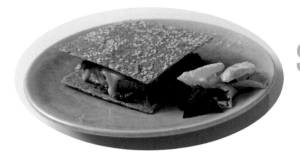

SNACKS, SIDES, AND TOPPINGS

ALFREDO SAUCE

INGREDIENTS

· 2 cups cashews (unsoaked)
· ½ cup pine nuts (or just use more cashews if you don't have pine nuts)
· 1 tablespoon lemon juice
· 3 cloves garlic
· 1¼ cups pure water
· 1 teaspoon dried thyme
· 1 teaspoon Celtic sea salt

DIRECTIONS

1. Place all ingredients in a blender and pulse, adding olive oil and water touch by touch until the mixture is smooth.
2. Pour, serve, and enjoy.

GUACAMOLE

INGREDIENTS

· 1 avocado
· 1 onion, finely chopped
· 1 bunch cilantro
· 1 lemon
· 1 teaspoon cumin
· Pinch of Celtic sea salt

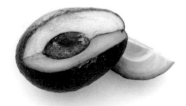

DIRECTIONS

1. Mash the avocado in a bowl.
2. Chop the onions and cilantro.
3. Mix onions and cilantro into the mashed avocado.
4. Juice the lemon and add the juice to the avocado mixture, to preference.
5. Mix in the sea salt and cumin to taste.

Option: Create a wrap with the guacamole using nori sheets (seaweed) or romaine lettuce leaves.

HERB PESTO

Great served over vegetable pasta or the Raw Pizza crust recipe on page 310.

INGREDIENTS

- 3 cups fresh basil leaves (or arugula, cilantro, lemon balm, marjoram, parsley, rosemary, sage, or young catnip)
- 5 cloves garlic
- 1 cup pine nuts or walnuts, soaked overnight
- ¾ cup extra virgin olive oil
- 1 teaspoon Celtic sea salt

DIRECTIONS

Combine all ingredients in a blender or a food processor and puree. Makes 4 to 6 servings.

JICAMA FRIES

INGREDIENTS

- 1 jicama, peeled and finely cut in thin, narrow strips
- A drizzle of olive oil
- 1 teaspoon chili powder
- 1 pinch Celtic sea salt
- 1 teaspoon nutritional yeast

DIRECTIONS

1. Chop the jicama into thin narrow strips.
2. Drizzle the olive oil over the pieces of jicama and dehydrate to desired softness.
3. Sprinkle the nutritional yeast, sea salt, and chili powder to taste.

KALE CHIPS

INGREDIENTS

- 2 cups kale, de-stemmed
- ¼ cup raw cashews
- 1 tablespoon coconut oil
- 1 teaspoon curry powder
- 1 teaspoon Celtic sea salt
- 1 tablespoon nutritional yeast

DIRECTIONS

1. In a food processor, mix all ingredients except the kale.
2. Rub the mix into kale and lay out to dehydrate in the dehydrator at 105° F.

LIVE VEGAN SOUR CREAM

INGREDIENTS

- 1 cup macadamia nuts, soaked
- 1 cup or less of pure water
- 1 clove of garlic
- Juice of ½ to 1 lemon
- 1 teaspoon Celtic sea salt
- 1 teaspoon sauerkraut (optional)

DIRECTIONS

1. Place everything except the water in the Vitamix or other blender, and then slowly pour in enough water to be able to blend at a high speed.
2. Continue to add more water until the dip is smooth and looks like sour cream.

NUT CHEESE

INGREDIENTS

- 2 cups macadamia nuts, soaked 4 hours (or another favorite nut, such as almonds)
- ½ cup pine nuts
- 2 cloves garlic
- 2 tablespoons fresh lemon juice
- 1½ cups water
- ½ teaspoon black pepper
- 2 teaspoons Celtic sea salt
- 1 teaspoon fresh basil

DIRECTIONS

1. Combine all ingredients in a blender or food processor and puree.
2. Place mix on a teflex sheet (a nonstick dehydrator sheet) and place in the dehydrator until most of the water is removed. (Makes 4 servings.)

Option: You can also add nutritional yeast or other types of herbs to suit your taste.

Can be served on vegetable pasta or pizza.

OLIVE PESTO

Serve over vegetable pasta or on dehydrated crackers.

INGREDIENTS

- ½ cup pitted, sun-cured black olives
- ¼ cup basil
- 1 tablespoon lemon juice
- 1 tablespoon extra virgin olive oil
- ½ teaspoon chili powder

DIRECTIONS

Combine all ingredients in a blender or a food processor and puree. Makes 2 servings.

RECIPE OF THE DAY: RAW POPCORN

This easy recipe is proof that living foods are fun! The popcorn does not have to be dehydrated to be enjoyed and often is eaten before the job is done anyway.

INGREDIENTS

- 1 head cauliflower
- ½ cup nutritional yeast
- ¼ cup olive oil
- Pinch of Celtic sea salt

DIRECTIONS

1. Chop the cauliflower florets into small popcorn-sized bits and put them in a bowl.
2. Add the nutritional yeast, salt, and oil to the bowl and cover the cauliflower completely with the mixture.

Option: You can dehydrate the cauliflower for up to 4 hours or longer for a more distinct popcorn texture and taste.

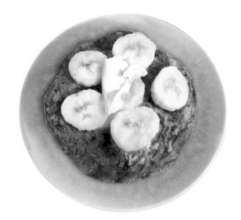

VEGAN BREAKFASTS

RECIPE OF THE DAY: **BANANA-TOPPED VEGAN PANCAKES**

This divine recipe is proof that health, beauty, and indulgence blissfully coexist. Feel free to try a gluten free ready-made flour mix and nondairy substitutes.

INGREDIENTS

- 1¼ cups almond or rice milk
- 1 tablespoon lemon juice
- 1 tablespoon vegetable oil
- 1 tablespoon maple syrup plus extra for serving (grade B has more minerals)
- ½ cup buckwheat flour
- 1 teaspoon baking soda
- ½ cup flour or flour mix, choice
- ½ teaspoon salt
- 2 bananas, thinly sliced

DIRECTIONS

1. Mix all wet ingredients in a small bowl.
2. Mix all dry ingredients together in a slightly bigger bowl.
3. Combine the wet to the dry and stir just enough to mix.
4. Heat a large nonstick skillet over medium-high heat.
5. Spoon the batter onto the skillet and cook for about a minute and a half or until the bottom side is golden brown and the top has small bubbles.
6. Repeat until you run out of batter, then serve with slices of banana and maple syrup.

COMFORTING WHOLE GROAT OATMEAL

INGREDIENTS

- ¾ cup whole oat groats, soaked overnight, rinsed, and drained
- ¼ cup buckwheat or short-grain brown rice, soaked overnight, rinsed, and drained
- 4 cups pure water
- Pinch of Celtic sea salt
- 1 tablespoon coconut oil (extra virgin, cold pressed)
- 1 tablespoon raw honey, coconut sugar, agave, or maple syrup
- 1 teaspoon cinnamon or maca powder
- Splash of vegan milk of choice (almond, rice, coconut, hemp, or soy)
- ⅓ cup goji berries or choice of dried fruit (optional)

DIRECTIONS

1. Boil water and salt, stir in oats and rice (which have soaked overnight), and bring down to a simmer.
2. Continue cooking on low heat, stirring often, until mixture is thick.
3. Serve hot with coconut oil, cinnamon, berries, sweetener, and a splash of nut milk.

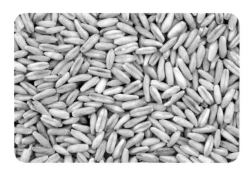

JUMPSTART CHIA BREAKFAST

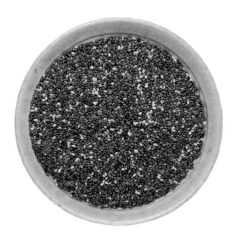

INGREDIENTS

- 3 tablespoons chia seeds, soak in fresh water 15 minutes to 8 hours for desired consistency
- 1 tablespoon of coconut sugar (or other favorite sweetener)
- 1 teaspoon vanilla or maca powder
- 1 Pinch of Himalayan or Celtic salt

DIRECTIONS

1. Presoak chia or stir in a bowl with water until it gels up.
2. Stir in remaining ingredients and serve.

Option: Add your choice of strawberries, mangos, blueberries, orange, papaya, or banana.

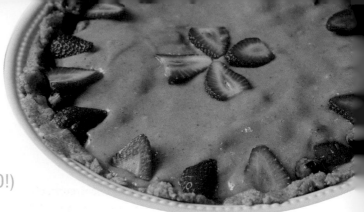

DESSERTS
(MAKE GREAT BREAKFASTS TOO!)

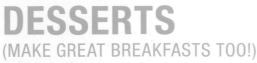

RECIPE OF THE DAY: **BUTTERSCOTCH PUDDING**

Indulgence and purity coexist in this blended treat. A delight for breakfast or dessert.

INGREDIENTS

- 1 cup dried apricots, soaked overnight in water (reserve soaking water for blending)
- 2 ripe peeled bananas
- 8 dates, pitted and soaked
- 1 teaspoon vanilla extract
- ¼ cup raw almond butter
- Hint of butterscotch extract if accessible

DIRECTIONS

Process in the food processor with an "S" blade. (4 servings)

CHIA PUDDING

INGREDIENTS

- 3 cups chia seeds
- 6 cups pure water
- 3 to 4 tablespoons maple syrup
- Cinnamon to taste (optional)
- Clove to taste (optional)
- Nutmeg to taste (optional)
- ½ chopped apple
- ½ cup chopped strawberries
- ½ cup blueberries

DIRECTIONS

1. Put the chia seeds in a bowl and soak. It takes about 10 minutes for the chia to absorb all the water, but leaving the water and chia to soak overnight is okay. Soaked chia alone is good for up to 2 weeks.

2. When the chia is gelatinous, add the chopped fruit and any desired flavorings (sweetener, spices, fruit, etc.). Mix well and serve!

Note: In general, soak chia seeds in 9 to 12 times their volume of water.

You can also make chia as a savory, salty, or spicy type of porridge. But the best taste is sweet.

Try it with cinnamon extract and chai spices or cacao nibs as well.

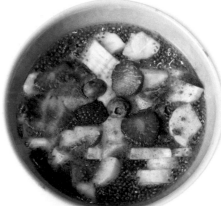

CHOCOLATE MOUSSE–DIPPED STRAWBERRIES

INGREDIENTS

- ¾ cup dates, soaked until very soft with pits removed
- 1 cup almond milk (raw, unpasteurized))
- ½ cup almond butter (raw, unpasteurized)
- 2 avocados
- ¾ cup cacao powder
- ½ cup raw honey, agave, or maple syrup
- Strawberries or your choice of fruit or nut

DIRECTIONS

1. Combine ingredients and blend or process until smooth.
2. Dip each strawberry, fruit, or nut of your choice in the chocolate mousse and place on plate or cooking sheet.
3. Refrigerate until slightly firm and serve.

COCONUT PUDDING OR PIE FILLING

INGREDIENTS

- The meat of 3 to 4 young Thai coconuts
- The water of 1 coconut
- 3 dates or 1 tablespoon agave or raw honey
- Pinch of Celtic sea salt

DIRECTIONS

1. Scoop out the meat of the coconuts.
2. Combine all the ingredients in the blender.

Option: For extra decadence, mix with UliMana Truffle Butter instead of sweetener.

LIVE CHOCOLATE PUDDING

INGREDIENTS

- The fresh meat of 1 Thai coconut
- 1 avocado
- 3 to 4 dates (soaked and pits removed)
- 2 to 3 tablespoons cacao powder
- 1 teaspoon cinnamon
- 1 teaspoon vanilla powder
- Pinch of Celtic sea salt
- 1 teaspoon chia seeds

DIRECTIONS

Combine all ingredients and blend until creamy smooth.

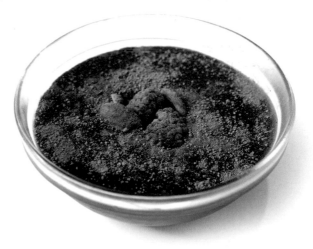

MORINGA BLISS BALLS

INGREDIENTS

· 1 cup walnuts (raw, organic)
· 1 cup dates
· 1 pinch Celtic sea salt or Himalayan pink salt
· 1 teaspoon to 1 tablespoon coconut oil (or olive oil, depending on your desired texture and consistency)
· 1 teaspoon vanilla powder (raw, organic)
· Optional: 1 teaspoon to 1 tablespoon raw cacao powder or 1 teaspoon to 1 tablespoon raw moringa powder

DIRECTIONS

1. Combine walnuts, dates, salt, coconut oil, vanilla powder, and (optional) cacao or moringa powder in a food processor and mix until ingredients bind like dough.
2. Empty contents into a bowl and with clean hands roll teaspoon-sized amounts of dough into balls and set on plate or cookie sheet.
3. Place balls in the fridge or freezer to firm, and serve.

Option: For extra bliss, roll balls in shredded coconut, cinnamon, spirulina, cacao, or your choice!

What are the health benefits of moringa? Scientific research confirms that these humble leaves are a powerhouse of nutritional value. Gram for gram, moringa leaves contain: seven times the vitamin C in oranges, *four* times the calcium in milk, *four* times the vitamin A in carrots, *two* times the protein in milk, and *three* times the potassium in bananas.

RAINBEAU'S GUILT-FREE STRAWBERRY PIE

INGREDIENTS—CRUST

· 2 cups macadamia nuts
· 1 teaspoon Celtic sea salt
· 1 teaspoon vanilla powder
· 1 tablespoon raw honey (or desired amount of dates)

INGREDIENTS—FILLING

· 1 banana
· 2 to 3 figs (or dates or prunes)
· 2 to 3 cups strawberries, sliced (or your choice of fruit)
· 1 teaspoon vanilla powder
· 1 tablespoon chia seeds
· 1 tablespoon raw honey (or use 2 to 3 tablespoons if not including figs, dates, or prunes)
· ¼ cup coconut water (or pure water)

DIRECTIONS

1. Combine crust ingredients in a food processor and pulse until the mixture binds like dough.
2. With clean hands, gather the dough and press evenly into your pie pan.
3. Then, as a base, lay out sliced strawberries so they are covering the breadth of the pan.
4. Next, blend the filling ingredients in a Vitamix or other blender, using more or less coconut water to reach desired consistency.
5. Pour filling over the layer of strawberries and decorate with a few more sliced strawberries on top. Voilà!

RECIPE OF THE DAY: **RAW KIWI-LIME COCONUT PIE**

This blended bliss combines the brightness of lime and kiwi with the satisfying creaminess of coconut and soaked nuts.

INGREDIENTS—CRUST

- 1 cup walnuts, soaked and rinsed
- 1 cup macadamia nuts, soaked and rinsed (or all macs and no walnuts)
- ¼ teaspoon Celtic sea salt
- 6 dates
- ¼ teaspoon vanilla (optional)

INGREDIENTS—FILLING

- 2 tablespoons Irish moss, soaked 12 to 24 hours and rinsed
- 1 fresh kiwi lime, skinned
- 1½ cup coconut water (young Thai coconut)
- ½ cup coconut meat (young Thai coconut)
- 1 ripe avocado
- ½ cup cashews or macadamia nuts (soaked and rinsed)
- ¼ cup raw honey, maple syrup, or agave nectar (to taste)
- 1 tablespoon fresh lime juice
- 1 teaspoon vanilla
- ⅛ teaspoon Celtic sea salt
- ½ cup coconut butter or coconut oil

DIRECTIONS

1. Combine raw crust ingredients in a food processor with the "S" blade and mix thoroughly. Remove and press into pie pan.
2. Chill or dehydrate for 5 hours.
3. Combine Irish moss and coconut water until smooth.
4. Gradually add remaining filling ingredients, blending until thick and creamy.
5. Pour into pan over prepared piecrust and chill in fridge.
6. When set, garnish with lime slices and serve. Skin and slice the kiwi to display internal ringed pattern of each slice.

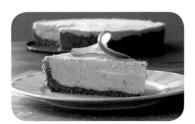

SIMPLE SWEET ALMOND BONBONS

INGREDIENTS

- 1 cup of almond flour (recommend brand: Divine Organics)
- 2 teaspoons maca powder (recommend brand: Divine Organics)
- 1 teaspoon grated orange or lemon zest
- ½ ripe banana
- 1 tablespoon coconut oil (recommend brand: Taste of Paradise)
- 1 teaspoon of sweetener (optional—I prefer organic raw honey)

Note: You can balance the taste of too much sweetener with a teaspoon of raw cacao powder.

DIRECTIONS

1. In a bowl, mix all ingredients with your hands and form into small balls. The amount of coconut oil needed may vary.
2. Refrigerate to solidify dough. Enjoy!

SHAKES, SMOOTHIES, JUICES, AND TONICS

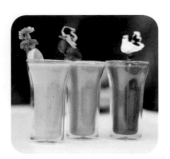

ACV TONIC

INGREDIENTS

- 3 cups pure water
- 1 to 3 tablespoons apple cider vinegar (unfiltered and unpasteurized)
- ½ to 1 whole lemon, juiced
- 1 to 2 tablespoons raw honey to taste

DIRECTIONS

Stir and enjoy this simple, super liver tonic.

ALMOND MILK

INGREDIENTS

- 1 cup almonds, soaked overnight and rinsed
- 1 quart of pure water
- 1 teaspoon raw honey or 2 dates, soaked

DIRECTIONS

1. Blend almond milk ingredients.
2. Strain through a nut milk bag, sprout bag, or strainer. Makes 1 quart.

Note: When making nut milk, save the pulp for making cheese. These same directions can be used for making cashew, hazelnut, sesame, sunflower, walnut, or pecan milk.

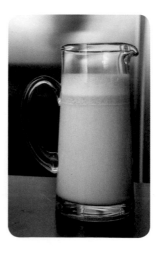

Option: Use leftover almond pulp in other recipes such as raw flour, pie crust, cookies, or flax crackers.

Option: Use hemp seeds in place of almonds to make Hemp Milk, a healthful nut and dairy milk alternative.

AMAZING MOJITO

INGREDIENTS

- Kombucha (lemon or regular)
- Lime
- Mint
- Raw honey

DIRECTIONS

1. Cut lime and mint and put in the bottom of your glass.
2. Add 1 spoonful of raw honey (according to your desired sweetness).
3. Mix lime, mint, and raw honey all together.
4. Pour in regular or lemon kombucha. Yes, amazing!

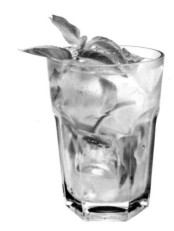

RECIPE OF THE DAY: BANANA ALMOND SHAKE WITH GINGER

This creamy goodness is simply Nirvana in a glass.

INGREDIENTS

- 1 cup almond milk (see recipe on page 330)
- 1 ripe banana
- 2 soaked dates
- 1 teaspoon vanilla extract (optional)
- 2 tablespoons almond butter (optional)
- 1 inch of fresh ginger

DIRECTIONS

Blend all ingredients and enjoy. (1 serving)

BLESSED DELIGHT TEA

INGREDIENTS

- 1 tea bag or 1 tablespoon loose-leaf holy basil (also known as tulsi)
- 1 teaspoon Shaman Shack Herbs 3 Immortals
- 4 cups of pure water
- ½ lemon
- 1 tablespoon raw honey, agave, or maple syrup
- Pinch of Celtic sea salt

DIRECTIONS

1. Cover holy basil in cup with an inch of cool water to protect the herbs.
2. Pour hot water and sweeten to taste.
3. Add coconut, rice, soy, or almond milk to your cup for a soothing latte.

CHAI TEA LATTE

INGREDIENTS

- 1 tea bag or 1 tablespoon loose chai mix
- 1 teaspoon ground cinnamon
- ½ teaspoon ground ginger
- ¼ teaspoon ground allspice
- 2 cups pure water
- 1 pinch of Celtic sea salt
- 1 cup vegan milk of choice (almond, rice, coconut, hemp, or soy)

DIRECTIONS

1. Cover chai tea in cup with an inch of cool water to protect the herbs.
2. Pour hot water and add in any of the spices you desire. Sweeten to taste.
3. Add your favorite vegan milk.

Option: If you want to give it the frothiness of a latte, you can put it in the blender for a few seconds.

Note: French press loose-leaf tea for a stronger brew.

CINNAMON DIGESTIVE SMOOTHIE

INGREDIENTS

- 1 peach or 4 apricots
- 1 whole orange
- 2 cups almond milk
- 1 teaspoon cinnamon
- 1 teaspoon vanilla extract (or powdered Madagascar vanilla)
- Pinch of clove
- Pinch of Himalayan or Celtic salt
- 1 teaspoon flaxseeds

DIRECTIONS

1. Remove the pit from the peach or apricots.
2. Peel the orange and remove as many seeds as possible.
3. Add all the ingredients to the blender and blend until creamy smooth.

Option: Add 1 teaspoon of Sunwarrior Ormus Supergreens to encourage optimal assimilation.

COCONUT BLAST

INGREDIENTS

- The meat of 1 young Thai coconut
- The water from the coconut
- 3 dates or 1 tablespoon of raw honey
- 1 teaspoon vanilla extract
- 1 teaspoon of psyllium husk powder, soaked flax, or chia seeds
- Small pinch of Himalayan or Celtic salt

DIRECTIONS

1. Scoop out the meat of the coconut.
2. Add to blender along with the rest of the ingredients. Blend and enjoy!

Option: To add a specific flavor, you can add your choice of strawberries, mangos, blueberries, oranges, papaya, or bananas.

COCONUT DELIGHT

INGREDIENTS

· 1 to 2 fresh young Thai coconuts
· 1 tablespoon coconut oil (unrefined)
· Pinch Celtic sea salt
· ⅛ cup cacao, moringa, or maca powder (optional)
· 2 to 3 dates or 1 tablespoon raw honey

DIRECTIONS

1. Crack open a fresh coconut and pour water into a blender.
2. Scrape the interior coconut meat with a spoon and add to the blender.
3. Add remaining desired ingredients to taste and blend until smooth.

RECIPE OF THE DAY: DEVA IN SEVA HARMONY TONIC

In Sanskrit, Deva means "divine being" and Seva is the spirit of selfless service. This tonic offers a toast to both of these aspects within you.

INGREDIENTS

· 1 to 2 apples
· 1 beet
· ¼ cup chopped or shredded purple cabbage
· 1-inch piece daikon radish
· 1-inch piece of ginger
· 1 handful blackberries and/or grapes (as in season)
· 1 teaspoon gotu kola (optional)

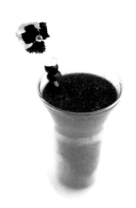

DIRECTIONS

1. Juice all of the ingredients.
2. Stir in gotu kola or your favorite superfood supplements.

GREEN CLEAN JUICE

INGREDIENTS

· 1 lime
· 1 handful kale
· 1 apple (Granny Smith)
· 1 cucumber
· 1 handful dandelion greens
· 1 sprig parsley
· 1 sprig cilantro
· 1 cup green grapes

DIRECTIONS

Put each of the vegetables and fruits above (or your favorites) through the juicer and combine.

Option: Stir in wheatgrass juice or HealthForce VitaMineral Green for added superboost.

HOT APPLE CIDER TEA

INGREDIENTS

- 4 cups of pure water
- 3 tablespoons apple cider vinegar (unpasteurized)
- ½ cinnamon stick
- 1 tablespoon raw honey, agave, or maple syrup
- Pinch of Celtic sea salt

DIRECTIONS

1. Boil water with cinnamon stick in pot.
2. Strain into mug filled with remaining ingredients. Stir and savor!

Option: Add coconut, rice, soy, or almond milk to your cup for a soothing latte.

LEMONADE

INGREDIENTS

- 2 tablespoons raw honey
- 4 cups pure water
- 6 lemons, limes, orange, or grapefruit

DIRECTIONS

1. Blend all together in a blender.
2. Garnish with mint sprigs. (Serves 2)

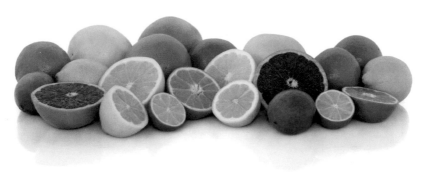

LIVE CHOCOLATE SHAKE

INGREDIENTS

- 2 to 3 cups raw almond or coconut milk (or pure water)
- ½ banana (optional)
- 1 handful strawberries (optional)
- 1 ripe avocado
- 1 tablespoon raw honey
- 2 to 3 tablespoons cacao powder
- 1 teaspoon cinnamon
- 1 teaspoon vanilla extract (or powdered Madagascar vanilla)
- Pinch of Celtic sea salt

DIRECTIONS

Combine all ingredients and blend until creamy smooth.

Option: Add 1 teaspoon of Sunwarrior Ormus Supergreens to encourage optimal assimilation.

RECIPE OF THE DAY: **LIVE DIVINE CHOCOLATE MACA SHAKE**

A heart-opening and hormone-enhancing celebration in a glass.

INGREDIENTS

· ¼ cup Brazil nuts (soaked and rinsed) or other raw nuts.
· 1 ripe avocado
· 1 semi-frozen banana
· 2 tablespoons raw honey or maple syrup (optional)
· 1 cup Brazil nut milk (optional: almond or coconut milk, or pure water)
· 2 to 3 tablespoons raw cacao powder
· 1 tablespoon bee pollen (optional)
· 1 tablespoon maca powder
· 1 teaspoon cinnamon powder
· ½ teaspoon Celtic sea salt

DIRECTIONS

Blend all the ingredients until smooth. Add cold or room-temperature water if needed to adjust to desired thickness (but do not add warm water or heat this recipe).

Option: Spice it up by adding Living Libations Immune Illume Hotberry.

RECIPE OF THE DAY: **MYSTIC MANGO SMOOTHIE**

A luscious antioxidant blend for the nourishment of eyes, skin, and soul.

INGREDIENTS

· ¾ cup fresh (preferred) or frozen blackberries
· 1 mango, pitted and chopped
· ⅛ cup goji berries
· ¼ cup pomegranate juice or coconut water (pure water is good too)
· 1 tablespoon cacao or coconut butter
· 1 tablespoon royal jelly or bee pollen
· 1 teaspoon maca powder (optional)

DIRECTIONS

Combine all ingredients, blend until smooth, and serve.

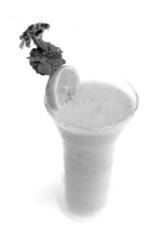

SUPER TONIC SMOOTHIE

Making a Super Tonic Smoothie can be nutritious and revitalizing.

INGREDIENTS

- 1 cup of organic yogurt (preferably nondairy)
- ½ ripe banana
- ½ teaspoon ginseng powder
- 1 tablespoon raw almond butter
- 1 tablespoon nutritional yeast
- 1 tablespoon maca
- 1 tablespoon tocotrienols

DIRECTIONS

Blend and enjoy!

SUPERBOOST SHAKE

INGREDIENTS

- 2 cups vegan milk of choice (almond, rice, coconut, hemp, or soy)
- 1 scoop Sunwarrior's Warrior Blend or quality protein powder of choice
- 3 tablespoons nut butter of choice
- 2 tablespoons maca (optional)
- 2 tablespoons cacao (optional)
- 1 teaspoon vanilla or cinnamon (optional)
- 1 tablespoon raw honey, coconut sugar, or 3 dates

DIRECTIONS

Blend ingredients together until creamy and smooth for a super boost of energy.

SUPERFRUIT SMOOTHIE

INGREDIENTS

- 1 mango or papaya
- ¼ cup goji berries
- ½ cup blackberries
- ½ cucumber
- 2 tablespoons aloe vera juice
- 2 tablespoons superfood powders or concentrates: noni, mangosteen (a tropical fruit grown primarily in Southeast Asia, containing anti-inflammatory, antimicrobial, antifungal properties), acai, durian, or other favorite
- 1 cup vegan milk of choice (almond, coconut, hemp, rice, or soy)

DIRECTIONS

Blend all together in a blender. Super invigorating. (Serves 2)

SUPERSTAR GLOW BEAUTY SMOOTHIE

A delectable beauty tonic to nurture your SuperStar Glow from the inside out!

INGREDIENTS

- 1–2 cucumbers
- 1 beet
- ¼ cup goji berries
- 1 cup grapes (as in season)
- ½–1 avocado
- 1 lemon
- 1 teaspoon Shaman Shack Herbs 3 Jewels

DIRECTIONS

Blend ingredients together until creamy and smooth to support your natural beauty.

WARM MACA MOCHA 'N' CINNAMON

INGREDIENTS

- 1 to 1½ cups hot water
- 1 tablespoon cacao powder
- 1 teaspoon raw honey
- ½ teaspoon maca
- Pinch of cinnamon
- ½ cup fresh almond milk

DIRECTIONS

Add all the ingredients in a blender or Vitamix and blend until frothy.

YERBA MATÉ LATTE

INGREDIENTS

- 1 tea bag or 1 tablespoon yerba maté (loose leaf)
- 4 cups of pure water
- 1 tablespoon raw honey, agave, or maple syrup
- 1 pinch of Celtic sea salt

DIRECTIONS

1. Cover yerba maté in cup with an inch of cool water to protect the herbs.
2. Pour hot water and sweeten to taste.
3. Add your favorite vegan milk.

Option: French press your tea for a stronger brew.

THE DOCTRINE OF SIGNATURES

A philosophy handed down through time by shamans, master herbalists, and visionary foodies, the Doctrine of Signatures states that whole, natural foods resemble the various parts of the body that most benefit from their use. As you prepare to stock your refrigerator and pantry with rejuvenating foods, consider the wonders of nature—and notice how she communicates with us through color, texture, and shape.

BODY ORGAN	FOOD	WHOLE FOOD SIGNATURE
Brain	Walnut	Looks like a little brain: a left and right hemisphere, upper cerebrum, and lower cerebellum. The wrinkles and folds of the nut resemble the neocortex. We now know that walnuts help develop more than three dozen neurotransmitters for brain function.
Eye	Carrot	Cross-section looks like the human eye—the pupil, iris, and radiating lines. Science shows that carrots greatly enhance blood flow to and functioning of the eyes.
Heart	Tomato	The tomato has four chambers and is red. The heart is red and has four chambers. Research shows tomatoes are indeed a pure food for heart and blood health.

BODY ORGAN	FOOD	WHOLE FOOD SIGNATURE
Mammary glands	Grapefruits, oranges, and other citrus fruits	Look just like the mammary glands of the female and actually assist the health of the breast and the movement of lymph in and out of the breast area.
Kidneys	Kidney beans	These actually heal and help maintain kidney function, and yes, they look exactly like human kidneys!
Pancreas	Sweet potatoes	Look like the pancreas and actually balance the glycemic index to positively affect diabetics.
Womb and cervix	Eggplant, avocados, and pears	Target the health and function of the womb and cervix of the female—each looks just like these organs. Research shows that eating one avocado a week balances hormones, sheds unwanted weight, and prevents cervical cancers. How profound is this? It takes exactly nine months to grow an avocado from blossom to ripened fruit. There are over 14,000 photolyctic chemical constituents of nutrition in each of these foods.
Testicles (and sexual libido)	Peanuts	These have a profound effect on the testicles and sexual libido. During the Middle Ages, peanuts were banned as a food for males by the church. Arginine, the main component of Viagra, is naturally occurring in peanuts.

BODY ORGAN	FOOD	WHOLE FOOD SIGNATURE
Penis	Bananas, cucumbers, zucchini	Each affects the size and strength of the male sexual organ. Yes, it's true!
Testicles, Sperm	Figs	Figs are full of seeds and hang in twos when they grow. Figs increase the mobility of male sperm and increase the numbers of sperm as well, to overcoming male sterility.
Ovaries	Olives	Assists the health and function of the ovaries.
Bones	Celery, bok choy, and rhubarb	Resembling bones, these foods specifically target bone strength. Bones are 23 percent sodium, and these foods are 23 percent sodium. If you don't have enough sodium in your diet, the body pulls it from the bones, making them weak. These foods replenish the skeletal needs of the body.
Body cells	Onions	Research shows that onions help clear waste materials from all of the body's cells. They even produce tears, which wash the epithelial layers of the eyes.
Blood cells and heart	Grapes	This awesome fruit hangs in clusters that resemble the heart. Each grape looks like a blood cell. Research shows that grapes are also profound heart- and blood-vitalizing food.

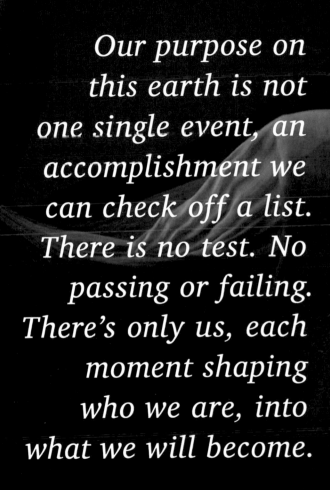

Our purpose on this earth is not one single event, an accomplishment we can check off a list. There is no test. No passing or failing. There's only us, each moment shaping who we are, into what we will become.

—CYNTHIA HAND

WHEN YOU
KNOW BETTER
YOU DO BETTER.

—MAYA ANGELOU

RAINBEAU'S READING ROOM

Welcome to my Reading Room! The following section offers a wealth of additional information that will not only help you to get the most out of your twenty-one-day cleanse, but also serve as a reference guide to support the choices you make about your food and health well into the future. In some cases, I am expanding upon ideas that we began to explore earlier, such as the importance of an organic, alkaline diet. In other instances, I'm addressing useful practices that can further augment your cleanse experiences, such as how to soak grains or how to self-administer an enema. One of the sections I think you will find especially helpful is Q&A with Rainbeau, where I answer a variety of practical questions that have arisen for superstar cleansers around the globe. May this compendium serve your greatest health for years to come.

GO ORGANIC

Did you know that organically grown foods contain 80 to 200 percent more vitamins, minerals, and other micronutrients than conventionally grown foods? Organic foods differ from conventionally produced foods in how they are grown, handled, and processed. And most conventionally grown foods are subjected to herbicides, pesticides, and other deadly chemicals.

When shopping for organic produce and other foods, it is important to note that the terms "natural" and "organic" are not interchangeable. You may see other words such as "free-range," "hormone-free," and "natural," but don't confuse these terms with the word "organic."

When buying organic produce, you should know that some produce is more protected from pesticides than others. For example, studies suggest that when a fruit or vegetable has an inedible skin, pesticides do not enter the edible portion of it. Conversely, some produce is very susceptible to pesticides. This produce forms a group called "the dirty dozen" and should *always* be bought organic. If you can't buy organic, try to reduce your consumption, or avoid the produce completely.

Here is the "dirty dozen" from a 2010 report published by the Environmental Working Group:

- Celery
- Peaches
- Strawberries
- Apples
- Blueberries
- Nectarines
- Bell Peppers
- Spinach
- Kale
- Cherries
- Potatoes
- Grapes (imported)

Please note: The USDA makes no claims that organically produced food is safer or more nutritious than conventionally produced food, particularly processed foods (i.e., organic cookies have nutritional value similar to the nonorganic variety). However, you can notice the biggest difference between organic and conventional foods when you buy fresh and frozen unprocessed produce (fruits and vegetables). It is also significant to note that if you can remove chemicals, toxins, and other free radical–producing substances from your diet, you will assist in accelerating your body's natural ability to heal.

For more detailed information on USDA organic standards, visit the USDA National Organic Program website: www.ams.usda.gov.

8 REASONS TO GO ORGANIC

In addition to the health benefits of eating organic food, there are reasons to buy organic that go beyond the quality of the food. Here are eight of them:

1. **Perfect water quality:** Water makes up two-thirds of our body mass and covers three quarters of the planet. Pesticides and other chemicals widely contaminate ground water and rivers and pollute our primary source of drinking water. Support companies that protect our water and other precious resources.
2. **Save energy:** Conventional farming uses more petroleum than any other industry. More energy is now used to produce synthetic fertilizers than to till, cultivate, and harvest crops. Organic farming is still based on labor-intensive practices such as hand weeding, green manure, and cover crops instead of chemicals.
3. **Keep chemicals off your plate:** Many pesticides approved for use by the EPA were registered long before extensive research had established the link between these chemicals and cancer and other diseases. Now the EPA

considers 60 percent of all herbicides, 90 percent of all fungicides, and 30 percent of all insecticides carcinogenic. A 1987 National Academy of Sciences report estimated that pesticides might cause an extra four million cancer cases among Americans! The bottom line is that pesticides are poisons designed to kill living organisms, and they can also harm humans. In addition to cancer, pesticides are implicated in birth defects, nerve damage, and genetic mutations. Let's pay attention to whether we are being part of the problem or part of the solution.

4. **Protect farm workers:** A National Cancer Institute study found that farmers exposed to herbicides had six times more risk than non-farmers of contracting cancer. In California, pesticide poisonings reported among farm workers have risen an average of 14 percent per year since 1973, and 100 percent between 1975 and 1985. Field workers suffer the highest rates of occupational illness in the state. Farm worker health is also a serious problem in developing nations, where pesticide use can be poorly regulated. Pesticides poison an estimated one million people annually. We could be indirectly killing people by choosing to support commercial farming that uses these types of chemicals on their workers.

5. **Help small farmers:** Although more and more large-scale farms are making the conversion to organic practices, most organic farms are small, independently owned family farms of fewer than a hundred acres. It's estimated that the United States has lost more than 650,000 family farms in the past decade. Organic farming is one of the few survival tactics left for family farms.

6. **Support a true economy:** Although organic foods might seem more expensive than conventional foods, conventional food prices don't reflect hidden costs borne by taxpayers, including nearly $74 billion annually in federal subsidies. Other hidden costs in conventional food production include pesticide regulation and testing, hazardous waste disposal and cleanup, and environmental damage. As an example, if you add in the environmental and social costs of irrigating a head of lettuce, its price would range between $2 and $3 a head. Organically grown vegetable crops give longer breaks to the soil to restore the vitamins and minerals that our bodies need.

7. **Promote biodiversity:** Mono-cropping is the practice of planting large plots of land with the same crop year after year. While this approach tripled farm production between 1950 and 1970, the lack of natural diversity of plant life has left the soil lacking in natural minerals and nutrients. To replace the nutrients, chemical fertilizers are used, often in increasing amounts. Single crops are also much more susceptible to pests, making farmers more reliant on pesticides. Despite a tenfold increase in the use of pesticides between 1947 and 1974, crop losses due to insects have doubled—partly because some insects have become genetically resistant to certain pesticides.

8. **Taste better flavor:** There's a good reason why many chefs use organic foods in their recipes—they taste better. Organic farming starts with the nourishment of the soil, which eventually leads to the nourishment of the plant, and ultimately our palates.

Lester Brown, founder of the Worldwatch Institute, has said: *We have not inherited the earth from our fathers; we are borrowing it from our children.* We must protect future generations through the food choices we make today.

For more information about organic food and farming, visit the online home of California Certified Organic Growers: www.ccof.org.

WE HAVE NOT INHERITED THE
EARTH FROM OUR FATHERS;
WE ARE BORROWING IT FROM
OUR CHILDREN.
—LESTER BROWN

UNDERSTANDING PH BALANCE

All biochemical reactions in the body can be expressed with a measurement of pH. pH stands for potential hydrogen, the degree of concentration of hydrogen ions in a substance or solution. Depicted by a logarithmic scale from 0.0 to 14.0, a lower pH suggests less potential for absorbing hydrogen ions (more acidity), while a higher pH means there is a greater potential for absorbing hydrogen ions (more alkalinity).

The pH in your body controls the pace of the body's biochemical reactions, including metabolic function and enzyme activity, by controlling the speed at which electricity moves through the body. More alkalinity creates more electrical resistance; thus electricity travels more slowly through higher pH. The opposite is true for acidity. Think: high pH (alkaline) = slow and cool, and low pH (acidic) = hot and fast.

The pH of your body is created through the foods you eat and the liquids you drink, and even in how you live your life. In today's world, people find themselves pressured to multitask, and they become stressed, exhausted, burned out, polluted, and quick to anger. In many ways, we are a society that is running hot and fast, living an acidic lifestyle. Fortunately, you do not have to be a victim of the world around you, because what you eat and drink will affect your body's pH levels. This can influence your body's electrical system, intracellular activity, and utilization of enzymes, vitamins, and minerals positively.

The ideal pH for the human body is about 6.4 (slightly alkaline) in order to build an alkaline reserve for acid-forming conditions such as stress, lack of exercise, pollution, or poor dietary habits. However, either extreme—being too alkaline or too acidic—can be detrimental to healthy body function. Most natural foods are alkaline by nature, but manufactured, processed foods are acidic.

Alkaline-producing foods include fruits, vegetables, sprouts, cereal grasses, and herbs. Examples of acid-forming foods are high-protein flesh foods (meat, fish, poultry, eggs), high sugar (refined sugars, processed desserts, soft drinks), high-fat and mucus-forming foods (dairy), low-complex carbohydrates (flour products, pasta, breads, most cooked grains, most beans, most nuts—except almonds), as well as coffee, tobacco, alcohol, drugs, synthetic vitamins, chemical additives, and preservatives.

Foods cause acidity in the body because they lack the oxygen and the enzymes (destroyed when cooked or processed) that are necessary for the food to be absorbed into the bloodstream. When the food is not absorbed, it is left to float as waste products in the bloodstream, raising acidity levels through autointoxication. In an effort to neutralize the internal acidity in an eternal search for homeostasis, alkaline minerals are stolen from our bones, tissues, and body fluids.

The key to regulating the body's pH is to balance essential nutrients from our daily dietary intake of food, generally making each meal 75 percent alkaline and 25 percent acidic. Though the proper ratio of acid and alkaline-forming foods can vary depending on our individual lifestyle, food preparation, chewing, genetics, exercise, and mental outlook, if you are prone to illness, infections, viruses, excessive mucus, or other acidic toxic conditions, you may benefit from a more alkaline diet.

In myself and with others, I have watched higher alkalinity turn bodies from stiff to flexible, rapidly creating an environment that is open and alive and accelerating the ability to go deeper into stretches and back bends. While an acidic environment might make you stronger, contracted, and even muscular, alkalinity seems to create an open and more expanded environment, so ultimately we want a combination of both. The problem is that most people spend the majority of the time in the more contracted state—experiencing a more contracted version of themselves—so doing this program supports that balance.

Acidity and Alkalinity in the Body

As I said before, the acid and alkaline balance is measured on a scale from 0.0 (acid) to 14.0 (alkaline). Neutral (neither acidic nor alkaline) is considered to be 7.0. While our stomachs contain stomach acid, the acid-alkaline state of the whole body can be monitored as well. This means taking into consideration the acid-alkaline balance of your muscles, blood, organs, and tissues (not just your stomach contents).

From the perspective of Chinese medicine, yin qualities are associated with alkaline, and yang qualities are associated with acid. Yin is cold, inclusive, gentle, magnetic, and passive—alkaline. Yang is hot, commanding, concentrated, fiery, and active—acid. Interestingly, alkaline elements attract negative charges where the positively charged ion (an electrically charged atom or molecule) *expands* to take electrons into its electric field (changing its charge to negative). Acid elements *contract* to give their negative charge away—just as Chinese medicine explains yin-yang characteristics.

Aside from keeping the body in homeostasis, or the balance that it seeks to maintain, there are some serious side effects that are caused by the body being either too acid or too alkaline.

When there is too much acidity in the body, there is an excess of hydrogen atoms, which can deplete oxygen by combining with the oxygen atoms to create water (H_2O). When less oxygen is available, lactic acid builds up. The system becomes even more acidic, and cellular function is diminished. Too much acidity can cause inflammation, puffiness, tissue tightness, and slowed brain function. Acidosis is a major contributing factor to drug addiction and is a breeding ground for cancer, diabetes, parasites, and immune deficiencies.

Signs of acidosis (overacidity) are craving coffee, alcohol, marijuana, cocaine and other drugs, stress headaches, anger and short temper, muscle stiffness and spasms, sinus congestion, irritability, lethargy, negative thought patterns, and itchy skin.

Foods may be acidic in composition, like lemons, but it is the food's effect on the body when it is metabolized that determines whether it is labeled acid or alkaline. In the case of lemons and other citrus fruits, these foods are actually quite alkalizing, although when they are pasteurized they have an acidic effect. Some foods that produce acid in the body are listed below:

ACID FRUITS

Cranberries (slightly), pineapple (if picked unripe), plums, prunes, strawberries

ACID VEGETABLES

Rhubarb, sauerkraut

ACID GRAINS

Barley, bread, flour products (pasta), kamut, oats, rice (slightly), rye, spelt, wheat

ACID NUTS AND SEEDS

Nuts (Brazil, cashew, hazelnuts, macadamias, pecans), oils, peanuts, seeds (pumpkin, sesame, sunflower seeds)

ACID ANIMAL FOODS

Cheese, chicken, crab, cream, duck, eggs, fish, ham, lamb, meats (all), milk, oysters, pork, turkey, veal

ACID MISCELLANEOUS

Alcohol amphetamines, beans (most, including adzuki, kidney, lentils, and navy; exceptions: lima and soy), candy, carob (slightly), chocolate, cocaine, coffee, curry, drugs, marijuana, morphine, pepper, sodas, sugar, tobacco, vinegar

ACID PRODUCING EMOTIONAL FACTORS

Anger, hate, negative thoughts, over-emotionalism, overwork, pollution, sleeplessness, stress, worry

Alkalinity occurs when there is less hydrogen in the body. Hydrogen-forming ions (or alkalis) are most prevalent in the body fluids and blood because cells tend to be more alkaline. Even the body's mechanisms help create alkalinity in the body; for example, the lungs contribute by removing carbon dioxide and bringing in oxygen. While maintaining a certain level of alkalinity is important, being overly alkaline is unhealthy.

Symptoms of being overly alkaline include: anxiety, excitability, spaciness, laziness, lack of ambition, always feeling cold, muscle spasms, slow recovery from injury, muscle tension and pain, low tolerance of stimulation.

Alkaline-forming foods, when metabolized, form alkalis (or bases in the body), leaving an alkaline "ash" residue. Even if the food is acidic in nature, this "ash," the product of metabolism, promotes alkalinity in the body. During digestion, the acids in lemon, for example, are oxidized into water and carbon dioxide to create an alkaline condition in the body. Some foods that produce alkalis in the body are listed below:

ALKALINE FRUITS
Apples, apricots, avocadoes, ripe bananas, cantaloupe, citrus fruits, dates, figs, grapes, guava, kumquats, lemons, limes, litchi, loganberries, mangos, all melons, mulberries, nectarines, olives, oranges, papayas, passion fruit, peaches, pears, persimmons, pineapples (ripe), plums, pomegranates, raisins, raspberries, sapote, watermelon

ALKALINE VEGETABLES
Algaes, artichokes, asparagus, string beans, beets, broccoli, brussels sprouts, burdock, cabbage, carrots, cauliflower, celery, collards, corn (fresh), cucumbers, dulse, eggplant, endive, escarole, garlic, herbs, horseradish, Jerusalem artichoke, kale, kelp, kohlrabi, lettuce, mushrooms, mustard greens, okra, onions, parsley, parsnips, peas (fresh), peppers, potatoes, pumpkins, radishes, spinach, spirulina, sprouts, squash (summer and winter), sweet potatoes, Swiss chard, tomatoes

ALKALINE GRAINS

Buckwheat, millet (Sprouted grains become more alkaline.)

ALKALINE ANIMAL FOODS

Acidophilus, bee pollen, butter, goat's milk, raw honey, mother's milk

ALKALINE MISCELLANEOUS

Almonds, coconut, garbanzos, lima beans, miso, mung bean sprouts, nutritional yeast, olive oil, soybeans, umeboshi plums (Japanese salt plums), vinegar

ALKALINE-PRODUCING EMOTIONAL FACTORS

Happiness, laughter, positive thinking, rest, sleep

Most people will find their health and well-being improve from becoming more alkaline. Even if your typical lifestyle tends to be rather acidic, there are a few simple steps you can take to become more alkaline:

1. Decrease animal foods, protein, fat, and sugar.
2. Eat more raw fruits and vegetables.
3. Drink alkalizing juices like cucumber, celery, and leafy greens.

If you have the more rare (but just as serious) overalkalinity, increase more acid-forming foods like nuts, seeds, fermented foods, garlic, onions, and cranberries in addition to exercising more.

Electrolyte minerals also help in balancing pH. Electrolytes are minerals (including calcium, lithium, magnesium, phosphorus, and potassium) that, when in solution, conduct electricity. If your body is either alkaline or acid, electrolytic materials will allow the excess charges an opportunity to express themselves, causing balance to restore.

Knowing the acidity or alkalinity of your foods and emotions encourages you to make good choices when preparing a meal or choosing the foods you want to consume for that day. If you have exercised frequently and have lactic acid buildup, choose more alkalizing foods or even lemon juice in water. Additionally, keep in mind that the emotions you experience while preparing these foods also impact the body—knowing how to make foods with confidence and happiness allows your body to feel happy and healthy.

I can literally see the difference between a body that is more alkaline or acid when someone is working out, practicing yoga, or even standing still. One of my teachers and colleagues, John Friend, describes the difference as "muscular" or "organic" energy. You can almost see *organic* energy moving out from one's core, expanding, giving, and sometimes being out of alignment and lacking boundaries, while *muscular* energy is moving in toward the center, contracting, being strong, and at times being stiff. Organic energy moves easily but can also be injured over time without your knowing that it's happening, and muscular energy has to work harder at moving but more easily maintains structure. Which type of energy best describes you? Can you see these energies in your friends? The goal is, of course, to have both and to have balance in both, resulting in alignment and openness. These are the inner and outer pulses of the core self that are balanced in the practice of *ra'yoKa* and other systems of yoga and fitness.

Practices that Shift the Acid-Alkaline Balance

- Whole grains and legumes (which are slightly acidic) can be soaked and sprouted (an alkalizing process) before cooking them.
- The digestive process begins in the mouth as voluntary action, and continues involuntarily after swallowing. This is why it's important to chew each bite thoroughly and avoid drinking with meals. Drinking with meals inhibits saliva (an alkaline and enzyme-rich fluid that helps neutralize food before it enters the stomach).
- Buy organic produce. It can be more alkaline than conventionally grown chemical- and pesticide-laden produce.
- Cook your foods less; gently steam vegetables or eat them raw, sprouting or soaking grains and legumes to eliminate enzyme inhibitors. This will create a more alkaline environment in which to digest your food.

THE ESSENTIAL NUTRIENTS

WATER
- Essential, major constituent of all body cells
- Removes waste from the body
- Eat foods with a high water content and drink lots of herb teas

FATS
- Concentrated source of energy
- Source of essential fatty acids
- Transport fat-soluble vitamins A, D, E, and K for use in cells
- Essential for proper brain function

PROTEINS
- Grow and repair body tissue
- Form the structure of body cells
- Maintain normal fluid balance
- Regulate body functions
- Produce antibodies to fight infection and disease

CARBOHYDRATES
- Main source of energy for all tissues, including the brain and nervous system
- Source of glucose for nerve tissues

VITAMINS
- Maintain body processes
- Support effective use of other nutrients
- Essential for normal physical and mental development

MINERALS
- Building materials for bones, teeth, and other tissues such as blood and nerves
- Regulate body processes
- Maintain normal fluid and acid-base balance
- We need all ninety-eight minerals to be perfectly healthy

TEN MORE REASONS TO GO RAW

For the uninitiated, eating a diet of primarily living foods might seem like a daunting task. However, there are many benefits of making the transition to raw food. In addition to the information outlined in chapter 3, here are ten more fabulous reasons:

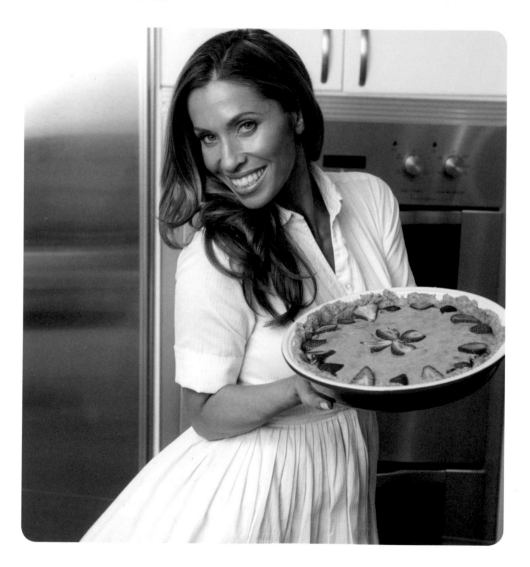

1. **Spiritual.** Living food promotes clarity and higher consciousness. A raw food diet helps people feel healthier emotionally and improves overall well-being and vitality.

2. **Environmental.** Fruits and vegetables require less land to produce than animal products. You save energy when you don't cook. Most of what gets thrown away can be composted back into the earth. In many countries, cooking fires contribute to deforestation.

3. **Flavor.** Flavor in raw food is vibrant, requiring fewer additives such as salt, oils, and sweeteners. There are more nutrients and fiber in raw food, and minerals are not leached out into the cooking water. Any recipe enjoyed cooked can be even better raw. An apple by itself is delicious. When baked, it then needs sugar, butter, and spices to be tasty.

4. **Beauty.** Raw food diets slow the aging process. You'll feel better, have more energy, and need less sleep. Bad breath and body odor go away. Eyes become brighter and voices become clearer. Skin and muscle tone improve.

5. **Save time.** Once you get into the flow of raw food preparation, you will spend less time in the kitchen. Many raw foodists ascribe to the "5-5-5 rule": No more than $5, five minutes, or five ingredients to prepare a meal. Please check out the YouTube video *Seven Minutes to Go Raw,* in which my mother makes seven raw dishes less than ten minutes!

6. **Nutrition.** There are more nutrients in raw food than cooked food. For example, some vitamins lose potency at 130° F (vegetables are steamed at 212°). The fat-soluble vitamins, A, D, E, and K, are destroyed in cooking. High temperatures can also cause the destruction of vitamin C and most of the B complex. Vitamin B1 loss from cooking can be from 25 to 45 percent. Loss of vitamin B2 can be from 40 to 58 percent. Cooking also disrupts the structures of DNA and the anticancer compound indoles.

7. **Health.** A raw food diet can help one overcome persistent ailments. The raw path has been used to improve the health of those with allergies, arthritis, asthma, high blood pressure, cancer, diabetes, digestive disturbances, diverticulitis, fibromyalgia, heart disease, weakened immunity, menstrual problems, multiple

sclerosis, obesity, psoriasis, skin conditions, and hormonal imbalances. It is more difficult to camouflage spoiled raw foods than cooked foods. Raw food requires more chewing, thus providing exercise for the teeth and gums.

8. **Energy.** Most people experience better work productivity and require less sleep when eating raw. Memory, concentration, and reason become sharper. The energy it takes to break down hard-to-digest foods can be rechanneled into other life activities.

9. **Economy.** Raw foods cost less, with most raw foodists spending between 25 and 80 percent less on food. A raw foodist spends lots less in restaurants, and raw food is nutritionally more dense and satisfying. A big spinach salad, when cooked, for example, becomes a measly, less satisfying portion. In addition, getting sick is expensive. Raw foodists spend money on good food and have the option of spending less money on doctors, hospitals, medicine, vitamins, and even recreational drugs!

10. **Easy cleaning.** Imagine never having to clean the oven! Dirty dishes can simply go in the dishwasher after a simple swoosh. No more baked-on grease requiring soaking and scrubbing! No more grease on your walls, stovetop, and ceiling.

LIVE RAW AND PROSPER.

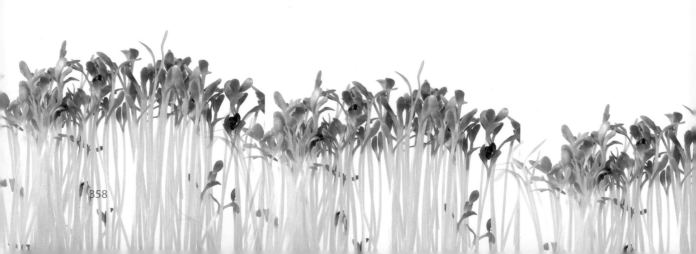

SPROUTING GUIDE

I love visiting Mom and eating sunflower sprouts off her tray of growing seeds, and one of my favorite dishes is her Sproutaroni (on page 312). Sprouted foods are the truest live food you can ingest. When a fruit or vegetable is taken from the earth or the mother plant, its life force begins to diminish. Sprouts, however, remain alive and continue to grow until the moment they are digested. The life force in sprouts is unparalleled by other living foods. In fact, sprouts are so full of life that some have been found still growing in such strange places as human lungs!

The process of sprouting is called germination, which makes the nutrients contained in seeds, grains, or nuts more bioavailable—unlocking the precious nutrient content. A sprouting seed breaks down its starches into simple sugars, and it breaks down its proteins into amino acids. It then uses both the sugar and amino acids to grow. As sprouts are rich with enzymes and all the nutrients and components of growth, they are powerful anti-aging and beauty foods.

It's important to note that many seeds, nuts, and other "sproutable" foods contain enzyme inhibitors like phytic acid that prevent the absorption of calcium, iron, and zinc. Ingesting these inhibitors can lead to an enlarged pancreas, digestive problems, and poor health. While cooking can destroy the inhibitors, it also destroys the enzymes within the foods. Sprouting, however, destroys the inhibitors but preserves the enzymes and nutrients within the food.

Here are several different plants that are easy to sprout:

- Clover
- Buckwheat
- Sunflower greens
- Fenugreek
- Mustard
- Radish

SPROUTING CHART

SPROUT TYPE	YIELD GIVEN	AMOUNT TO USE	SOAK TIME	TIME TO HARVEST	SPROUT LENGTH	SPECIAL INSTRUCTIONS
Alfalfa*	7:1	2 Tbsp.	8 to 12 hours	3 to 6 days	1 to 2 inches	None
Amaranth	1.5:1	⅔ cup	Do not soak	2 to 4 days	¼ inch	Rinse and drain 4 to 6 times per day for faster sprouting.
Buck-wheat	1.5:1	⅔ cup	20 to 60 minutes	1 to 3 days	Length of seed	Do not over soak. Rinse until water runs clear. Rinse and drain 3 to 6 times a day.
Clover	7:1	2 Tbsp.	8 to 12 hours	3 to 6 days	1 to 2 inches	None
Garbanzo	2:1	½ cup	8 to 12 hours	2 to 4 days	Length of seed	None
Lentil	2:1	½ cup	8 to 12 hours	2 to 4 days	Length of seed	Rinse red lentils until water runs clear.
Millet	1.5:1	⅔ cup	6 to 10 hours	1 to 5 days	$\frac{1}{16}$ to ⅛ inch	None
Mung	2:1	⅓ to ½ cup	8 to 12 hours	2 to 5 days	1½ to 3 inches	Sprout in darkness. Rinse often.
Oats	1.5:1	⅔ cup	30 to 60 minutes	1 to 3 days	Length of seed	None

SPROUT TYPE	YIELD GIVEN	AMOUNT TO USE	SOAK TIME	TIME TO HARVEST	SPROUT LENGTH	SPECIAL INSTRUCTIONS
Radish	5:1	3 Tbsp.	6 to 12 hours	3 to 6 days	1 to 2 inches	None
Rye	1.5:1	⅔ cup	6 to 12 hours	2 to 3 days	Length of seed	None
Sunflower	1.5:1	⅔ cup	1 to 4 hours	1 to 5 days	¼ inch	Rinse until water runs clear. Rinse and drain 2 to 6 times per day. Use within a week of sprouting.
Wheat	1.5:1	⅔ cup	6 to 12 hours	2 to 3 days	Length of seed	None

See caution regarding alfalfa sprouts and canavanine on page 362.

Note: Wheatgrass (compound word) refers to trays of wheatgrass grown indoors, whereas wheat grass (two words) refers to the outdoor variety. In mild climates, wheat grass can be grown outdoors in locations that are sunny but protected against direct sun from 11 a.m. to 3 p.m., when the sun's rays are most intense. This outside-grown version is far less likely to have mold than the store-bought version. Those who are prone to candida should consider getting tested for sensitivity to either type before consuming regularly.

IF YOU HAVE WATER TO THROW AWAY, THROW IT ON A PLANT.

—OLD HINDU SAYING

While you can eat any sprout, there are some sprouts that require extra concern. While mung beans and lentils are healthful and easy to sprout, many beans and alfalfa are not great sprouting choices. Beans do not play a major role in the live foods lifestyle because they are difficult to digest. When sprouted, beans still contain lots of starches that are not completely transformed into simple sugars. These partially converted starches make your body work harder to convert them into a usable form.

Caution: Alfalfa sprouts contain canavanine, which is an arginine analogue. Arginine is an amino acid that has many beneficial effects, but may be implicated in replication of the herpes virus (this is still being studied). Canavanine is designed to deter animals from eating the plant and is central to the plant's survival mechanism. So it is best to avoid alfalfa sprouts until further research is conducted, or unless you are sure the sprouts have been given ample time to pass the stage when canavanine is highest. Also, be mindful that some sprouts can get moldy, so pay attention and compost them if this happens.

TRAY SPROUTING FOR GRASSES

The tray method works best for barley, buckwheat, kamut, rye, spelt, sunflower, and wheat (for wheat, use the hard red berries, not soft wheat). One pound of seeds will make about four pounds of grass. It is best to get your seeds in the fall, because autumn is when they are at their peak freshness. Store the grain in a sealed container to keep out rodents, and store the container in a cool, dark location.

First, soak one-half cup of seeds in one cup of water (or enough water to more than twice cover the seeds). Soak your seeds for twelve hours or overnight. Next, prepare a tray filled with about five-eighths inch of growing medium. Growing medium can be organic potting soil or a combination of equal parts Canadian sphagnum peat moss and organic untreated soil. You can also use black humus from the woods (including leaf mold and the black earth underneath). A bit of kelp can be added to the soil to bring additional minerals inside the potting. Whatever growing medium you choose, the soil should be light and airy.

Spread the seeds out on the tray of dirt without piling them on top of one another. The soil needs to be kept moist, so keep the tray in the basement or cover it with plastic for the first few days to conserve moisture. In very dry climates, you may need to place a wet paper bag over the seeds. When the sprouts are about two inches high, remove any covering and place the tray near a sunny window. Three hours of sunlight daily is adequate, although more light will speed the growing process. (If the grasses are pale, they are not receiving adequate sunlight.) Water your sprouting grasses only once a day.

When the sprouts are eight inches high (about one week to twelve days), it's time to harvest them. Using scissors or a serrated knife, cut the sprouts as close to the surface of the soil as possible (many of the sprouts' nutrients are concentrated close to the soil). After the harvest, the roots of the grass will remain, and if you keep watering the tray, you will be able to obtain a second harvest. However, the sprouts of the second harvest will not be as nutritious as those of the first.

When the grasses have been harvested, compost the contents of the tray, which will be filled with grass roots. Adding a few earthworms to the mixture will facilitate breakdown.

Sometimes mold forms on the seed portion of sprouting grasses. It might look like white cotton, and will become grayer as it matures. Do not confuse mold with the young cilia hairs on the rootlets. Mold is most likely to form during hot, humid weather. It can also result from excess watering or inadequate spacing between plantings. Mold does not make the grass unusable; just wash it off the plants after harvest.

If flies are attracted to the mold, just vacuum them up as best you can. If mold turns out to be a chronic problem for you, you can prevent it by soaking seed for twenty-four hours in the refrigerator. Make sure you drain the sprouts and rinse them well. Also, allow the seeds to sprout for twelve hours before placing them in the soil. This said, if the sprouts do not feel fresh and clean and like they would beautify your system, simply compost the goodness and help grow more minerals for future crops.

SUPERSTAR SPICES

When making dishes, incorporate different spices and herbs to give your food a more exotic flavoring. Indian, Thai, and Vietnamese foods use a wide variety of flavors to enhance their taste. Here are some of the more popular cuisine styles and the herbs that transport the taste to the unique spot of international deliciousness you want to imitate.

- **Mexican:** coriander, cilantro, cumin, chili powders (cayenne, chili), paprika
- **Indian:** curry, turmeric, fenugreek, coriander, cumin, cayenne, clove, cinnamon
- **Creole:** sassafras, cayenne
- **Thai:** lemongrass, ginger, cilantro, cayenne, basil, kaffir lime
- **Italian:** basil, oregano, thyme
- **French:** parsley, sage, rosemary, thyme
- **Moroccan:** cumin, paprika, cinnamon, cilantro, pomegranate juice
- **Dessert spices:** clove, nutmeg, cinnamon, vanilla, cardamom, and cacao

When incorporating spices into your foods, if you find you have been either too zealous with the spicing, or perhaps a little too cautious, follow these simple adjustments.

- Start your recipe with less seasoning and water because you can easily add more. It is much harder to "subtract"!
- If you've oversalted or overspiced a dish, you can either make a new batch *or* make another batch completely unsalted and unspiced and mix the two together to hopefully neutralize the flavoring.

- Try to correct oversalted food by subtracting salt from every other part of your meal to balance it out.
- Add a little salt to your sweet dishes and add a little sweet to your salty dishes.
- When cooking, and especially sautéing, I always use dried herbs with a pinch of Celtic sea salt to season the food. Before serving, I'll add some fresh herbs that will still burst subtly in the mouth in an aromatic way.

Great accents for live food dishes can be both decorative and aroma-therapeutic! Add nature's healing plants as beautiful, healing additions to your dishes. There are so many different ways to season a dish while healing your body at the same time. You can include:

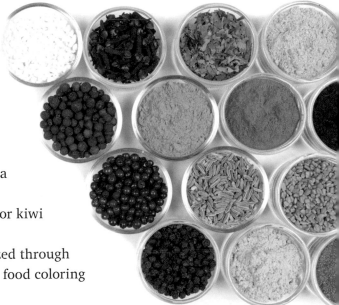

- Rose flower petals
- Rosemary sprigs
- Lemon or other citrus peels
- Edible flowers (borage flowers are bright and look like blue stars)
- Lavender or dandelion can be especially lovely
- Seeds and nuts like almonds or walnuts (poppy or sesame seeds for a layer of depth)
- Fruit like strawberries, blueberries, or kiwi for color
- Nut cream or frosting can be squeezed through cloth to create shapes and trim (use food coloring in nut creams for extra flair)

LET THY FOOD BE THY ART AND EXPRESS
YOURSELF THROUGH IT.

FIVE FLAVORS THEORY OF TRADITIONAL CHINESE MEDICINE

1—Sour

TASTES	Sour indicates the presence of acids (citric, malic, ascorbic acid).
ELEMENTS	Wood feeds Fire and grasps Earth.
FOODS	Sour is present in vinegar, lemons, berries, and any citrus fruit.
BODY	Liver and Gallbladder
EMOTIONS	Anger, creativity, and depression
REMEDIES	Creative activities like art. Herbal master Michael Tierra says art is "toxic discharge," which according to Traditional Chinese Medicine relates to an imbalanced Liver meridian.
CONCERNS	If a person has a troubled liver, they generally exhibit this with an addictive personality. Many people with liver troubles are actually very creative people who need to express themselves.
SUPERSTAR GLOW HABIT	Start every day with half a lemon in a glass of hot water to support the liver. Start the day with a Liver Kick or simply with water, lemon, and/or apple cider vinegar (with or without raw honey) for seasonal support for this hard-working organ.

2—Bitter

TASTES	Bitter flavor indicates that alkaloids are present. Alkaloids end in "ine" or "in": for example, cocaine, morphine, mescaline, and caffeine.
ELEMENTS	Fire creates Earth and melts Metal; Fire can "burn out of control" and "burn through a lot of resources," though it possesses the gift of speech.
FOODS	Bitter is present in green leafy vegetables like kale and arugula.
BODY	Heart and Small Intestines
EMOTIONS	Joy and lack of joy, tumultuous, high-drama marriages, divorce, depression, rehab stints
REMEDIES	More positively, bitter flavor opens the heart to compassion. This can be seen with chocolate and its theobromine. Antiseptic herbs like goldenseal and echinacea are bitter tasting; therefore, you can know they are strong medicine.
CONCERNS	Bipolar depression can be associated with the Fire element burning out of control.
SUPERSTAR GLOW HABIT	Americans get most of their bitters and alkaloids from coffee and chocolate. Try to integrate other bitter flavors into your diet.

3—Sweet

TASTES	Sweet indicates the presence of carbohydrates.
ELEMENTS	Earth produces Metal and contains Water (also Air).
FOODS	Starchy foods like carrots, apples, and grains. The ideal source of sweet is nature's, like the sweet from fruits, raw honey, nuts, roots, sweet potato and winter squash, and mother's milk.

BODY	Stomach and Spleen
EMOTIONS	Sympathy and obsession
REMEDIES	Balance your sugars: Overconsumption of sugar puts the body into immune system overdrive, producing a "high" when white blood cells are released. Some experts believe that imbalanced blood sugar levels set the stage for addictive behaviors.
CONCERNS	Diabetes or hypoglycemia (precursor to diabetes). In this culture, sugar is essentially a legal drug for kids. Two hundred years ago, the average American ate four pounds of sugar per year. Today's average is 152 pounds of sugar per year per person!
SUPERSTAR GLOW HABIT	"Full sweet" like that of refined sugar is sweet without minerals or other flavors. Sugar cane and sugar beets have the presence of full sweet, but processing these foods into sugar turns the sweet into a highly addictive flavor and substance. Instead, blend fresh produce into smoothies, maintaining fiber, which helps slow down sugar absorption. (*Note: Juicing can be high glycemic because the process removes fiber.*)

4—Spicy/Pungent

TASTES	Pungent foods or spicy foods indicate the presence of essential oils.
ELEMENTS	Metal condenses Water and cuts Wood.
FOODS	Garlic, ginger, cayenne, and thyme
BODY	Lung and Large Intestine
EMOTIONS	Grief and self-expression. Think about the spicy/pungent onion and its ability to make us cry. The flavor of onion helps us release unshed tears.
REMEDIES	Pungent foods are warming and improve circulation.

CONCERNS	Spicy/pungent foods can be strongly medicinal but can have the counter effect when used in excess.
SUPERSTAR GLOW HABIT	Explore the power of essential oils through aromatherapy or herbal infusions like ginger and thyme.

5—Salty

TASTES	Salty foods indicate the presence of minerals.
ELEMENTS	Water nourishes Wood and extinguishes Fire.
FOODS	Stinging nettles; sea vegetables like kelp, dulse, and nori; earthy foods like roots; and the obvious salt.
BODY	Kidney and Bladder. Kidney governs hair, teeth, and bones. Traditional Chinese Medicine considers the kidneys (and the corresponding Kidney meridian) to be the root of life.
EMOTIONS	If there are problems with the heart, there are often problems with kidney or liver. The emotions associated with salty flavors are fear and willpower. The emotion of fear can be seen in children wetting the bed, indicating insecurity or trauma.
REMEDIES	The kidneys like warmth. A good health exercise is to rub the kidneys up and down 36 times in each direction. Allow sunlight to shine on the back, or lie on a heating pad.
CONCERNS	Though salty foods indicate the presence of minerals, most table salt is heated to 1400° F and the minerals are removed and sold to vitamin companies. The salt is then bleached white to create a more appealing look.
SUPERSTAR GLOW HABIT	The color that nourishes the kidneys and Kidney meridian is black—anything very dark like chia seeds, black sesame seeds, seaweed, and dark leafy greens

28 BEAUTY RITUALS

FOR YOUR MEGAWATT GLOW

Throughout the twenty-one-day cleanse, you likely made a little extra time for self-care and pampering. Maybe you gave yourself that pedicure on Day Three, or walked barefoot on the ground on Day Fifteen. Or you might have given yourself a facial treatment and acupressure massage on Day Twenty and then enjoyed the "head-to-toe glow" dry brushing and bath extravaganza by the end of Week Three. Another possibility is that you are preparing for the cleanse by reading the entire book first and were particularly drawn to this section because you know that the benefits and rewards for prioritizing beauty are ample … and you are right. Throughout the entirety of the cleanse, there is an ongoing dance that takes place: as you take care of your body, you soothe your soul; as you make time for your emotions and your spirit, your body reflects the loving care. As you take care of yourself during these four weeks (including your re-entry and integration week), you are creating a new template for the days and years to come—days of health, days of exuberance, and yes, days of beauty.

In addition to the suggested beauty disciplines offered earlier in the book, here I'm offering twenty-eight more beauty rituals for turning up the dial to your glow. As you read them, notice which ones resonate with you right away, write them into your calendar as sacred appointments with yourself—and re-solve to try them all!

1. **The Feet.** In Chinese medicine, the feet are regarded as maps of the body, our connection to the earth, and the Hindus consider the feet to be sacred. If you live near sand dunes or a beach, one of the best ways to exfoliate your feet is to walk barefoot in the sand. Or you can buy an organic foot scrub and give yourself an at-home footbath. Work on spreading your toes and bringing awareness and intelligence to the part of the body that is farthest from your brain.

2. **The Eco-Pedicure.** After a footbath, paint your toenails using nontoxic, natural polish purchased at your local health food store. Or get a luxurious pedicure by trading with a friend or simply going to a nail salon. Lavish your feet with praise, and acknowledge them when you bring them to your face during yoga practice. If you have any problem nails (toenails or fingernails), eat foods high in silica, such as seaweed, green leafy vegetables, celery, and unpeeled cucumbers.

3. **Care for the Ankles and Legs.** People often regard their ankles and legs as being too thin or thick. When was the last time you had a little "quality time" with them, thanking them for the mobility they provide? As you spread and open the feet as recommended above, you energize the ankles and legs. Throw an ankle and leg party the next time you're in the bath or shower, remembering to exfoliate, wax, moisturize, and celebrate.

4. **The Knees.** Your knees are especially important because they bear a lot of weight. This part of the body carries a great deal of stress, especially if the hips are tight. Massage your knees with coconut oil while chanting your mantra of the day.

5. **The Upper Legs.** Also known as the quadriceps, the upper legs consist of the hamstring muscles and side hips, which are the strongest, largest muscles of the body. These muscles are the powerhouses for the rest of the body, affecting metabolism as well as endurance. Strengthening these muscles can burn body fat and increase our stamina for everything we do in life. During your next yoga session, on your next walk, or while dancing around your home, mindfully place your attention on your upper legs ... knowing that a little attention reverberates with a lot of strengthening love.

6. **The Bikini and Groin Area.** This intimate area of your body deserves and needs loving and enthusiastic attention too. Grooming and pampering with options like waxing or highlighting with lemon juice and sunlight offer opportunities to commune with the elements, bringing *sun* and *salt*

and *water* to this part of us that is normally hidden from view. Turn your grooming session into a visualization practice as well, putting your awareness on the first chakra, the subtle energy center at the root of your body. Notice what thoughts, feelings, images, or sensations arise as you do this.

7. **The Hips.** The hips are the largest joints in the body and need special care. Avoid sitting in a chair with one knee crossed over the other, as this constricts the flow of energy. Massage the hip area with quality oils, and take time to scrub with salts and a loofah. Most importantly, utter positive words to your hard-working hips and let old criticisms get sloughed off with your cleansing salts.

8. **The Navel and Solar Plexus.** Also affectionately called the belly button, the navel is where digestion begins. It is already thanking you for the high-fiber (fruits and vegetables) way of eating that you're committed to during the cleanse. If constipation or other digestive issues arise, either as a temporary occurrence or more chronically, colon hydrotherapy is often beneficial for alleviating these problems. Probiotics, such as acidophilus products, are excellent for digestion and repopulating the system with friendly bacteria. A gentle massage also helps. Try this: Place your left hand on your right side and go up, across your abdomen, and then down, moving in the same direction as your large intestine (in a clockwise path) and connecting to what's there. This will assist with digestion and metabolism. This area is the home of the third chakra (the chakra of the radiant gem). The color that we want to visualize here for balance is yellow. The element is Fire.

9. **The Kidneys.** The Kidney Rub is one of the Tibetan Five Rites, a system of exercise and rejuvenation that dates back at least 2,500 years. It's performed on the backside of the body, right underneath the lowest ribs. Make a fist and rub up and down in a quick motion thirty-six times to nourish this vital area that governs your hair, passion, and fearlessness in the world.

10. **The Heart.** On Day Nineteen of the cleanse, we focus on the heart in a direct way, honoring this vital organ that is the sacred symbol of the pulse of life. If we close down and don't protect ourselves in healthy ways, we are faced with depression, anxiety, and life-threatening problems such as heart disease. Keeping the shoulders integrated and in alignment helps the heart remain available and open. Apply lavender and rose essential oils to the chest and heart area. Wear comfortable, natural fiber undergarments, which allow the skin to breathe. This area is the place of the fourth chakra … the heart chakra.

11. **Your Crown of Glory.** It is best if hair isn't stripped of its oils by washing it too often. Many hair stylists recommend shampooing every four to five days, conditioning the ends. Use conditioners often and brush beautiful oils such as olive, coconut, or jojoba through the hair regularly. You can also use shea butter for deep conditioning treatments. These oil treatments can occasionally be left on overnight. Eat foods such as seaweed, black sesame seeds, green leafy vegetables like kale, and raw sunflower and pumpkin seeds to help the hair grow stronger and faster. This area is the home of the seventh chakra (the crown chakra), our connection to our higher selves, so take care to massage the scalp to stimulate and increase circulation.

12. **The Body as a Whole.** In chapter 4, we devote some quality time and attention to the power of dry brushing and bathing to restore and refresh (see Superstar Skin: Finding Your Head-to-Toe Glow on page 274). Here we turn our attention toward the nitty-gritty, you could say: the beautifying properties of oatmeal and Epsom salts. First, soak in a soothing bath of fresh herbs or teas, or add ten drops of essential oils, which are healing and antibacterial. Try peppermint for energy, grapefruit to stimulate the movement of blocked energy in fat cells, chamomile to relax, and eucalyptus to purify. Including Epsom salts in addition to the essential oils is the best for tired muscles. If you have psoriasis or generally sensitive skin, raw oatmeal tied into a washcloth and placed in the tub is soothing, softening, and calming to the skin. Avoid getting overheated; if you feel faint, splash your face with cool water. Adding a bath pillow, candlelight, a bowl of washed grapes, and organic juice or wine are favorite touches of mine.

13. **Turn Things Upside Down.** At work and at home, find places where you can take short breaks to put your feet *up*. Use a wall, a chair, or even your desk, and breathe, breathe, breathe. This will increase circulation, aid digestion, help prevent varicose veins and wrinkles, and improve your overall mood. Ultimately, you will get more done if you take small breaks and invite the nourishment of your blood, lymph fluid, and chi (life force energy) to circulate freely.

14. **Let Nature Relieve Your Stress.** There is nothing like the power of nature to wash away tension and stress and restore energy and perspective. Take a walk around your neighborhood, a hike in nature, a bike ride around town, or a swim at the lake (or other body of water). Take time to watch the sun set and feel your inner glow warming up.

15. **Soul Relief.** How many times in your life have you heard that the eyes are the windows to the soul? They are, most definitely, portals of our deepest self. So cry when you need and want to. Pain and suffering in your body and mind are released through crying, which in turn clears the soul. So let it go, let it flow, and allow yourself to be free and in the present.

16. **Positive Thinking Matters.** Have you heard the saying that "energy flows where attention goes"? Place your superstar focus of attention on what you like about yourself, such as your eyes, skin, hair, body, teeth, hands, or legs. Positive affirmations offer a way to bring your thoughts and feelings into focus to generate more of a good thing … and self-love is a very good thing.

17. **The Beauty of Being Responsible.** It's worth considering that taking responsibility for your choices and actions is a kind of internal beauty treatment. Being proactive, creative, resourceful, and emotionally honest is a recipe for inner peace and outer radiance.

18. **Releasing Fear—Expanding Consciousness.** Unraveling some of the knots of fear that we all deal with is another unsung beauty practice. Years of doubt, stress, and anxiety can melt away when we open up to receive

guidance from our higher consciousness. There are many ways to go about this, but one of the most elegant ways is to *ask* for guidance. "What do I need to know, see, or understand to release this fear and open up?" You can ask for insight and solutions to come through your dreams at night or as signs during your waking hours. Another effective practice is to write first thing upon rising in the morning, invoking a pure flow of consciousness. Write down your feelings, thoughts, desires, and goals. Write down how you aspire to be that day, and the people you would like to come into contact with. By writing things down, you give them power and a place of solid reality. Write, write, and keep writing ... it's writing for beauty!

And finally ... Ten Fast-Track Tips for Boosting Your Beauty and Joy

19. **Healing Music.** You can feel in your bones that music is healing on a deep cellular level, right? Unleashing emotional inspiration, the universal language of sound and music has a way of quickly connecting us with all that is beautiful, in ourselves and in the world.

20. **Nourish Your Mind.** Since you're constantly receiving and filtering input from our information-abundant world, it's important to consciously choose to feed your mind with beauty. Make it a practice to fill your mind with beautiful literature and art. Expand your creative potential.

21. **Touch the World.** Travel can be so uplifting and healing. Visit special places such as hot springs, mountain resorts, and spiritual grounds. Actively look for new places that provide rejuvenation and healing.

22. **Try a Thai Massage.** Let someone put you in yoga poses, stretch and rock your body, and encourage you to let go. It's like getting a month of facials.

23. **Watermelon for a Day.** A day of eating only watermelon is extremely cleansing, detoxifying, and nourishing.

24. **Lemon Liver Tonics.** If there is a river that runs through this book, it is a steady stream of water and lemon, with occasional flows of apple cider vinegar, raw honey, and cayenne. A happy liver is one of the great pathways to beauty.

25. **Restorative Yoga Poses.** Restoratives are long holds in yoga postures with little effort but lots of support. With the help of a wall and some blankets, blocks, and straps, your internal organs are profoundly nourished, quieting the mind and erasing tension from a furrowed brow. You can take restorative classes and/or learn a few of the poses and do them at home.

26. **Sexual Healing.** Sexual pleasure with closeness, care, awareness, and aliveness creates a sanctuary of beauty that transforms every corner of our lives. When people need help reviving or maintaining a healthy sex drive, I recommend trying the supplement *HotRawks* by Raw-Nation.

27. **Sleep In.** Some things need no explanation. ☺

28. **Raw cacao.** Edible, beautifying bliss.

INTRODUCTION TO COLON HYDROTHERAPY

There are countries where colon hydrotherapy is one of the first protocols that is applied when one becomes sick. This cleansing remedy began in ancient Egypt and India, with records of its use dating back to 1000 to 2000 BCE. Throughout much of Europe today, as well as in the field of Ayurvedic medicine that has been embraced in West, it's recognized that a healthy body and optimal immune system depend on a healthy intestinal system, which includes both the small and large intestines. Although colon hydrotherapy directly addresses the large intestine, it powerfully affects one's overall health by taking pressure off the liver and kidneys and releasing deep emotional holding patterns.

Colon hydrotherapy is a true healing art. In my own case, having colonics has helped me heal years of constipation, irritable bowel syndrome, acne, food allergies, mood swings, and other ailments, especially by allowing me to address the emotions the were underlying those imbalances. Colon hydrotherapy literally and figuratively helped me move stuck emotions and restore emotional flow.

Think about how often we have "eaten" our emotions and stored old wounds that we weren't ready or able to process. Addressing these layers of emotions is one of the reasons that the word "therapy" is so applicable to the art of colon hydrotherapy. In addition to the physical cleansing, it helps us access parts of ourselves that need love and that will benefit from releasing old anger, undigested hurt, and a backlog of tears. It's like you've been cleaning your house by simply throwing everything in the garage. Hidden from view, that mess grows out of control and can eventually become a serious health hazard.

If colon hydrotherapy is new to you, my goal is to give you the information you need to inspire you to try it. If you have already taken advantage of this protocol, my aim is to *re*-inspire you so you can take your healing process even deeper.

Water carries oxygen, and we want the entire body to breathe freely—especially those areas and organs that process the most and work the hardest. As the water removes the waste buildup, stress is washed away and lightness returns. It's exciting to note that in relation to yoga practice, this will help with back bends, handstands, and other inversions.

More on the Physical Benefits of Colon Hydrotherapy

The interior of our colon has enough surface area to cover a tennis court. As we move toward purifying our system, hydrotherapy can assist in the removal of accumulated wastes and blockages that contribute to bloating, constipation, nausea, food cravings, fatigue, headaches, and hemorrhoids. In the context of this twenty-one-day cleanse, it's important to know that colonics and enemas are excellent ways to alleviate many of the negative detoxification symptoms that are associated with cleansing and relative to the digestive tract.

I passionately recommend colon hydrotherapy sessions, especially while cleansing. This goes back to the idea of nurturing yourself while you are going deeper into purifying your body. This is also about supporting your body system so it can restore *itself* to optimal, vibrant function.

Conditions that often respond well to colon hydrotherapy

- Acne
- Allergies
- Arthritis
- Asthma
- Attention deficit disorder
- Body odor
- Brittle hair
- Brittle nails
- Cellulite
- Chest pain
- Chronic fatigue
- Cold hands and feet
- Colitis
- Constipation
- Excess weight
- Fibromyalgia
- Headaches
- Hypertension
- Irritable bowel syndrome
- Joint aches
- Memory lapses
- Mouth sores
- Multiple sclerosis
- Muscle pain
- Nausea
- Peptic ulcer
- Pigmentation
- Poor posture
- Pot belly
- Seizures
- Skin rashes
- Spastic colon
- Toxic environmental exposure
- Toxic occupational exposure

Important Message: If any of these conditions apply to you, check with your health care provider to explore whether colon hydrotherapy can be done at home or at a clinic. Although my suggestions are based on benefits that I have personally experienced and seen with my friends and clients, what is most important is that you do what is appropriate for you. See a licensed, board-certified practitioner for information and possible contraindications.

ENEMA INSTRUCTIONS

In serious wellness clinics such as the Ann Wigmore Institute or the Optimum Health Institute, at weight loss facilities like WE CARE, or in the Ayurvedic detoxification practice of Panchakarma, colonics or enemas are practiced up to twice a day. I recommend ideally doing some type of colon hydrotherapy once a day during Week Three of this program.

While colonics can be a significant factor in healing and rejuvenating, they aren't for everyone. Whether your economic situation, schedule, or anything else prevents you from engaging in colonics, there are other potent options—with the next best being enemas. An enema is more like a do-it-yourself hydrotherapy session. Enema bags are not very expensive and can be used more than once. This is a more personal, cost-effective, and schedule-friendly alternative.

What you will need:

- A clean enema bag
- Distilled water
- A towel
- Some time and privacy (having the bathroom or another space all to yourself for a while)
- Candles, incense, relaxing music
- In addition to good water, you might also opt to add chlorophyll, a few drops of an antibacterial essential oil such as peppermint, coffee (but not at night-time), yerba maté, and/or some olive oil
- A little bit of coconut or olive oil for lubrication

Steps for administering an enema:

1. Schedule about a half hour for your enema during a time when you think you can hold the water in for at least five minutes and eventually longer—aiming for ten, fifteen, and even up to thirty minutes (which is recommended by the yogis).

2. You can get creative with your time too. I like to stand on my head for a while when I do mine.

3. Warm your distilled water slightly on a stove. Or, if you're using de-acidified, organic coffee, mix with water so it's not too hot. As indicated above, water can also be mixed with chlorophyll, olive oil, or a couple of drops of an essential oil. Whichever liquid solution you choose, the temperature of the liquid needs to be tolerable—lukewarm to room temperature. So be sure to stick a finger in the water to test it; if it's too hot for your finger, it's definitely too hot for your colon.

4. Fill the enema bag (or bucket) with your liquid, and then close or clamp it shut, checking to see if the water or solution comes out of the tube and into the sink.

5. Position the bag about three to four feet high so it will be higher than the tube, allowing the liquid to flow with the pull of gravity.

6. Lay nice cozy towels on the bathroom floor and make a space where you can be comfortable.

7. Light some candles, play some beautiful relaxing music, and perhaps light some clearing, nonsynthetic incense. If necessary, post a "do not disturb" sign on the bathroom door, but it would be good to let anyone living with you know that you're taking some personal time for yourself so that you can relax and not worry about being interrupted.

8. With the help of your breath, relax and let go. In the tranquil and harmonious atmosphere that you've created for yourself, use this time as an opportunity to meditate and allow your body to rest and open.

9. Position yourself on your left side and put lubrication (the raw organic olive or coconut oil) on the enema tube (the part with one opening). Have as much as a cup of oil on hand to make insertion easy.

10. Open your mouth and breathe as you insert the tube inside. The mouth is directly connected to the anus, and they both need to receive the experience for optimal benefit from this ancient healing art.

11. Gently release the tube and allow the water to flow in until you feel too full to take in any more water. You may want to clamp the tube and pause until your muscles relax and you can take in more, or clamp and just take a break. *Note: If necessary, you can get off the tube, release the liquid into the toilet, clean yourself, and then finish the rest of the water.*

12. Eventually you will be able to take in the whole amount of water while lying on your back, massaging any tight spots in your body. Or you can do a little yoga—inversions and twists are particularly good during an enema, but the important thing is to be comfortable.

13. Finish on the toilet until you are fully done releasing. It may come in waves, so be patient and listen to your body ... and choose to let it all go.

14. Finally, take a cleansing shower and warmly acknowledge yourself for this act of self-care. Once you are *completely* clean, if you would like to linger with the healing waters for a while longer, you can follow with a peaceful bath.

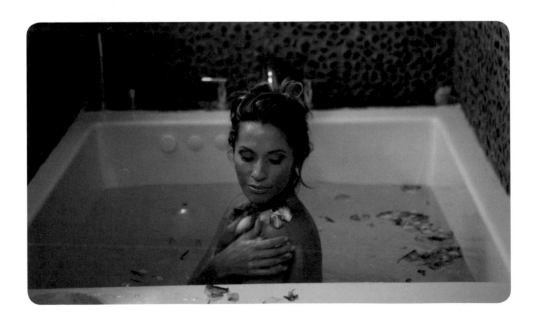

Q&A WITH RAINBEAU

FREQUENTLY ASKED QUESTIONS

Q: Do I wait twenty minutes after drinking the Liver Kick before having anything else?

A: Yes.

Q: I am really struggling with a bloated stomach, especially while cleansing. How can I alleviate this embarrassing issue?

A: First, if you are drinking soda, which hopefully on this program you're not, please switch to kombucha, coconut kefir (nondairy), or, better yet, a glass of water with a teaspoon of apple cider vinegar and the juice of half a lemon. The carbon dioxide in soda is something that the body is trying to get rid of with each inhale, so swallowing it whole can be confusing. That in addition to the sugars and synthetic sweeteners … it's just not the best. Ginger or peppermint teas also work wonders to ease bloating and stomach upset.

Q: Where do you get your protein?

A: I'm glad you asked! The word protein means "to come first." Protein is made from amino acids and contains nitrogen as the distinguishing element, as well as carbon, hydrogen, and oxygen. Protein is needed for tissue growth and repair and the formation of blood cells, antibodies, enzymes, hormones, and neurotransmitters. It is a source of food energy and helps in the water-electrolyte balance of the body.

Though Americans get plenty of protein, disease is rampant. Amino acids (there are twenty-two, eight of which must be obtained from outside sources) start being destroyed at 118° F and are virtually all deactivated by 160° F. Cooking causes the proteins to coagulate and become denatured. This makes proteins less digestible and more inflammatory. Cooking food to slightly under 200° F causes leukocytosis, where leukocytes (white blood cells) that would be used to attack a foreign substance are called in to help digest food. The renowned Max Planck Institutes (comprising nearly eighty research organizations under that umbrella, doing groundbreaking work in life science research) have found that even small increases in protein consumption can decrease the body's ability to transport oxygen, which can be a factor in cancers. After we eat a cooked protein meal, white blood cells increase by as much as 600 percent. This signals that the immune system is trying to maintain homeostasis. The Max Planck researchers have discovered that a person only needs half as much protein as previously believed when protein is consumed in its raw state. When eating raw or living foods, the need for protein decreases from about 70 grams daily to approximately 35 grams daily. When life is very stressful, the need for protein is increased.

Protein digestion uses up about seventy percent of its caloric content. Proteins are broken down into amino acids through an enzyme catalyzing process called proteolysis, usually with the help of hydrochloric acid. Excess protein can overload the lymphatic system's ability to cleanse itself. An excessively high-protein diet can contribute to heart disease, high blood pressure, arthritis, gout, kidney disease, osteoporosis, and liver and prostate disorders.

The media encouragement to eat more dairy, eggs, and meat is fueled by those industries that want you to buy their products. Though these foods are high in protein, they are also high in fats and represent the captivity, suffering, and exploitation of animals. Certainly humankind survived off animals during many times of hardship and necessity, but that practice is no longer needed for most people. As was outlined earlier in the book, eating lower on the food chain exposes one to less herbicide and pesticide residue. Also, consider the strength and power of oxen, racehorses, and gorillas—all of whom eat a vegetarian diet.

There is some protein in all foods. Protein is present in the nucleus of almost every cell of every life form on earth, in the form of DNA.

Complete vegetable proteins include: Alfalfa, almond, buckwheat, clover, garbanzo, lentil, millet, mung bean, pumpkin seeds, quinoa, sesame seeds, soy foods, sunflower greens, green leafy vegetables, and most fruits. All nuts, except filberts, are complete proteins, containing an average of ten to fifteen percent protein.

Other good protein sources include: Apricots, avocados, bananas, beans, bee pollen, berries, blue-green algae, broccoli, brussels sprouts, cabbage, carrots, cauliflower, cherries, chlorella, coconut, collards, corn, cucumbers, dandelion greens, dates, durian, eggplant, sprouted grains, grapes, green beans, green leafy vegetables, hemp seed, kale, lettuce, maca, melons, mustard greens, okra, sun-cured olives, oranges, papayas, parsley, peas, peaches, pears, peppers, seaweeds, spinach, spirulina, sprouts, summer squash, sweet potatoes, tomatoes, turnip greens, sprouts, watercress, and zucchini.

Vegetables have a higher percentage of protein per calorie than fruit (about four times as much of their total calorie content). On average, fruits have about as much protein as mother's milk. Fruits contain protein in amounts from four to ten percent of their total calorie content. Here are a few examples of the amount of protein in foods based on total calorie content:

- Almonds—12 percent
- Broccoli—45 percent
- Buckwheat—15 percent
- Cabbage—22 percent
- Raw honeydew—16 percent
- Kale—45 percent
- Pumpkin—15 percent
- Spinach—49 percent
- Walnuts—13 percent
- Watercress—84 percent
- Zucchini—28 percent
- Seaweed—5 to 30 percent, depending on type

Q: I am so hungry even after eating a raw food meal. What can I do about that?

A: Be sure to eat as much as you want and get as much liquid fat as possible—olive oil, coconut oils, soaked nuts, and avocado. It *is* a struggle if you are used to waiting to eat until you're starving or don't prepare enough food ahead of time. If you're still hungry, eat more live foods. It's hard to overeat live foods. *Whatever you do, do not go hungry, leaving room for the temptation to fill yourself back up with empty calories.* My best tip is this: prepare your meals *the day before* … even if you think you'll have time the next day. Preparing in advance doesn't necessarily mean combining the ingredients (you want everything as fresh as possible anyway). Instead, it means choosing a recipe and laying out the ingredients, bowls, utensils, and anything else you'll need for putting it all together in the morning. It will be worth it! You don't want to be half dazed and in a hunger craze, just staring at the cupboard wondering what in the heck you can do with the things inside. Think of it this way: preparing ahead of time will leave you feeling grounded, peaceful, and empowered.

Q: What about irradiated nuts and seeds? Are they still considered raw?

A: Most cashews, even though labeled "raw," are heated. Most pecans are heated, and so are American almonds. Therefore, the nuts and seeds to use during this cleanse are walnuts, pine nuts, Brazil nuts, Spanish almonds, macadamia nuts, sunflower seeds, and pumpkin seeds. The best nut butters are made by Rejuvenative Foods or Artisana, although they are pricey. I have not yet figured out how to make them on my own without overheating, but most raw nut butters on the shelves have actually been heated to the point of destroying the enzymes.

Q: Both my acupuncturist and my Ayurvedic practitioner react strongly when I mention my exploration of living foods due to a valid opinion that cooked food is better for the digestive "fires."

A: *Great question!* I understand this school of thought; I have worked with many Ayurvedic and Chinese medicine practitioners myself and have several friends and family members practicing these healing arts. Usually they start asking me for advice when they get food poisoning or feelings of depression. My baseline starting point is that I like to look at things holistically and consider everyone's points of view and ultimate goals. We are all here to learn from each other, and I respect and look for the truths in all things. Whether it's the paleo, blood type, vegan, macrobiotic, high-protein (Atkins), calorie constriction, lemonade fasting, South Beach, or Skinny Bitch diet, or Chinese medicine or Ayurvedic way of eating, there could be a time when one of these programs or paths is for you.

However, when you communicate with a holistic practitioner about live foods and do so with some education and knowledge, they will hopefully admit that live foods are cleansing, hydrating, and healing for a body that is burdened with inflammation and a build up of toxins.

Regarding the digestive fires: in reality, with live foods, *we do cook*—we are just not using *fire* to kill those vital enzymes. In effect, we cook through soaking, sprouting, fermenting, and even blending. While breads and unsoaked nuts can be slightly harder to digest than fresh ones, soaked nuts and seeds in moderation are usually digested well. Plus, nothing is harder to digest than the moldy, yeasty, glutinous, refined paste we find in most processed foods. Imagine looking at your liver and colon with X-ray vision after eating something like French fries or even a turkey burger as opposed to mineral-rich, leafy greens—then begin to make food choices from that place.

I have deep respect for Ayurveda. My godmother is an Ayurvedic doctor, and I was trained in the art, having lived with her as a teen. There is actually a great deal of compatibility between Ayurvedic cleansing programs and my living foods cleanse, in that live foods are common to both for purposes of cleansing and boosting the availability of digestive enzymes. The use of healing herbs can also be incorporated to ensure that the digestive fires are stoked.

Traditional Asian medicinal doctors love live foods. My mom (Brigitte Mars) studied and taught this art for many years and is a master herbalist. She and I both recognize the essential elements of yin and yang that operate within our bodies and all around us, and we understand that live foods are a vital aspect in balancing those energies. Even she resisted the "live food" diet until she saw that menopausal complications, wrinkles, cellulite, and health problems nearly vanished from her maturing body.

To sum up, for people who are experiencing deficiencies or low digestive fire or who may be very sick, juicing, fermenting, sprouting, and blending foods can greatly facilitate digestion. For those who need to cook foods because their digestion is not strong enough at this point, I recommend lightly steamed vegetables and foods that digest more easily, like quinoa and soups. However, this should not be a ticket to live off meat and grains, which are by far more challenging to assimilate and absorb.

A final thought on this topic: make sure you take your digestive enzymes!

Q: Why am I still so tired? Shouldn't my energy be increasing by now?

A: You may be tired because you are still detoxing. Chemicals, toxins, and previously unprocessed waste can leave us feeling tired while they're on the way out. This is an important aspect of preventative medicine; we need to give our bodies time and rest in order to heal, cleanse, and return to our natural state—healed, loved, balanced, refreshed, and clear.

Q: Is organic miso considered okay for Week Two and its focus on live foods?

A: Yes, miso is a live, fermented food. When preparing the hot water, make sure that it's not boiling so that it doesn't kill all the natural probiotics in the miso. Use warm water.

Q: What does "a day in the life" look like for Rainbeau when on a 100-percent live food diet?

A: Given that I am such a lover of being a "flexitarian" and enjoying the cuisines of the world, I usually kick my plan into full gear right before an on-camera job. Here is a typical schedule for me on a really good day (you'll notice that it looks a lot like the at-a-glance planners during Weeks One through Three):

- 6:30 a.m.—Wake up and spend quality time with my husband, doing our private yoga, and breathing techniques.
- 7:00 a.m.—One of us juices lemons and oranges for a Liver Kick, softening the taste bud shock with strawberries or raw honey.
- 7:30 a.m.—In all honesty, drinking yerba maté is a regular ritual for me. I find it a good catalyst for other herbs entering my bloodstream, so I often use tea with ginger and mint as the hot water that goes into the French press with the yerba maté.
- 7:45 a.m.—I really cannot get enough of thermogenic herbs! They give me the feeling of being warm from the inside out, and I imagine them healing through heating up any old residue. One of my favorite ways to eat them is by having soaked chia seeds with cinnamon, a little nutmeg, vanilla, fresh almond milk, and a touch of salt and raw honey. My daughter likes this too and has her own, simpler version. Often times, both she and my husband, Michael, grab a mama chia and go.
- 8:00 a.m.—Drive Jade to school. We communicate about absolutely everything. It's my philosophy thats kids are smarter then us, with fewer walls, so if they can start learning now, before they unlearn, they can surpass us, which is the aim. I alternate my training and yoga schedule, some days training in the morning and other days in the afternoon. Admittedly, sometimes I have to strait to work, depending on the project.
- 8:30 a.m.—Get some writing done and take care of errands.
- 10:00 a.m.—Company meeting time; go to an audition or some type of shoot; or work with my acting coach.
- 10:30 a.m.—Get more tasks done: conference calls, handle deliverables, etc.

- **11:30 a.m.**—I have a beauty shake that includes things like papaya, mango, almond butter, almonds, ginger, almond milk, and superfoods like maca, tocotrienols (not raw), MSM, raw honey, and cinnamon.
- **2:00 p.m.**—Warmed tortilla soup with *caliente* spices in a coconut base. I know; even my acupuncturist doesn't like my intake of spices. But I just love them.
- **3:15 p.m.**—Pick up Jade and take her to Kids Yoga, gymnastics, or dance.
- **4:00 p.m.**—Hit the mat and practice for two hours while Jade does homework and waits for me outside the yoga room.
- **6:00 p.m.**—Perhaps two big bowls of miso soup made from a seed cheese and water with fresh cilantro. Family dinner time. Our dinner will often be something like kale salad, corn tamales, tacos, burritos, or gluten-free pasta or pizza. They will actually try pretty much everything I make and call me a great chef! We sometimes go out to eat or attend an event. I also have salads, shakes, and raw desserts as part of a glowing beauty regimen. We love the raw pies and they are great to make, because we can eat them for breakfast too.
- **7:00 p.m.**—I alternate what's next with the activities listed from 7:30 on. I might go to a class: I am currently in a course called Landmark, for self-development and transformation, and I study acting. I attend a lot of charity events and music concerts at the Hollywood Bowl and other venues. These all typically last until 10:00 p.m. or later, so my schedule changes.
- **7:30 p.m.**—Sometimes it's a relaxing bath. I love to drink tea and water in the bath … ultra hydration.
- **8:00 p.m.**—Dance, read, write, draw, clean, and organize life for the next day.
- **9:00 p.m.**—Tuck in and kiss my daughter good-night.
- **10:00 p.m.**—Go to sleep to restore and rejuvenate for a bright new day. This is quite honestly a dream day. It doesn't always work out that I get to bed at this time, but I love it when it does.

Q: What about hormones? Which foods are nourishing and balancing for hormones?

A: Cacao can be a helpful tool, as it is high in antioxidants and is a bitter cardio tonic. But it's easily overdone, and its stimulating nature doesn't work for some people. Maca has a highly nourishing effect on the hormones (in women and men) and the entire endocrine system, including the thyroid and adrenals. It is a member of the cruciferous family, and therefore a close relative of rutabaga and turnip. I am currently taking iodine for a hypothyroid condition stemming from teenage abuse of chemicals and alcohol. It's important to get tested to find out what your hormone condition is. And if synthetic hormones are prescribed, be forewarned that they are often derived from pigs. Perhaps this is necessary and perhaps not. However, you might try gentler substances first and see if your body will once again start producing what it needs for balance. It is good to grow in our understanding of our bodies by becoming observers, like the scientists who examine their environment, the foods they eat, the thoughts they think, and the emotions they allow themselves to feel and those they stifle. Understanding can lead to compassion, and compassion can lead to better choices and greater healing.

In general, I believe that most hormonal concerns can be improved by supporting liver function. It is the liver that helps break down hormones. For more information on foods and herbs to increase and balance hormonal levels, please check out Brigitte Mars's book *The Sexual Herbal*.

If you haven't had a menses cycle in two years, it might be wise to get a check up. I have, however, seen good results with Gaia Herbs Vitex Elixir (accept no substitutes). Taking it consistently for six months has often been helpful to reestablish the moon cycle. Also, please try my Level Orange *ra'yoKa* download or the series from the virtual teachers training to understand and create harmony in this area of your body (go to www.rainbeaumars.com to access downloads).

Q: Help! I am plagued by cravings and it is sabotaging my desire to move forward with the program.

A: Okay, here are several things you can do to stop cravings:

- Take a dose of herbal bitters.
- Be sure to get adequate raw protein and fats.
- GTF chromium: 200 mcg four times daily can help reduce cravings.
- Spirulina with its high content of phenylalanine also reduces cravings and satisfies appetite.
- Green drinks help eliminate cravings, as they are very alkalizing.
- Rotate the colors of foods you eat to diminish cravings.
- Take an aromatherapy bath, have a luxuriously long phone call with some-one at a distance, or read for enjoyment.
- Write down all your temptations, as suggested during certain days of the cleanse.
- Eat avocados for PMS-related cravings.
- Craving salt may indicate a need for more minerals. Instead of potato chips, eat seaweeds, high-mineral foods such as Celtic sea salt, and raw cacao.
- Eating celery diminishes sweet food cravings.
- If you strongly crave fats, eat avocados. Add some nuts. But balance them with lots of leafy greens, celery, and cucumbers.
- Drink cardamom tea or smell cardamom.
- Smell jasmine essential oil.
- For cooked chocolate cravings, take ten deep inhalations of essential oil of cinnamon several times daily.
- Desiring something sweet, creamy, or carbohydrate rich is often about a need for warmth and nourishment. Drink some fennel tea or take ten deep inhalations of fennel essential oil.
- Wanting potato chips and salty, crunchy foods may indicate anger and frustration.
- When craving stimulants, which may indicate feeling dull or depressed, play upbeat music or drink some ginger or peppermint tea.
- Put a wedge between you and the craving. Do something else. If you are still craving a food, eat it and observe how you feel.

Q: What do I do when it is winter in my part of the world? It's freezing outside, and I am having a hard time with cold foods as I am already COLD!

A: Winter is naturally a time to build rather than cleanse. It's true that it is much easier to do aspects of this program in a more moderate climate or specific season. At the same time, given the holiday season and its many temptations to fall asleep and neglect one's health, it can also be one of the best times to customize a cleanse. Who doesn't want to begin the new year with a hot, best-version-of-yourself figure, radiant face, and great health? So be diligent, intelligent, and modest—and "keep that glow going" in all seasons. Shine an inspiring light on your cold and out-of-shape (and probably pasty) family, friends, and coworkers. Be an example that might inspire them to get on track as well. Make modifications and adapt the program to work for you. For example, you can make sure to have the Liver Kick tonic more often and/ or consider staying with Week Two's live vegan plan during Week Three as well, or simply stick with the easy-to-follow Week One plan for three weeks. Create the plan that works for you and your current goals.

Warm yourself with hot herbal teas and warming foods such as ginger, cinnamon, garlic, cayenne, and red- and orange-colored veggies. I also suggest lots of slightly warmed, blended soups made with warming foods, like blended carrot-ginger soup. Miso soup is also great with seaweed. Experiment with blending vegetables into soups. Wear warming colors like reds and oranges (including warm-colored socks). And remember to take warm baths. I must add that even in sunny California, I would be really sad without my luxurious baths. And no matter where I travel around the world, I make sure I have a bathtub, as warming baths keep my body relaxed and my practice flowing.

Q: I'm feeling dehydrated, but I am drinking more water than usual.

A: For hydration, put a pinch of Celtic sea salt into your water and try eating more seaweed. You may need more minerals. This can sometimes happen when you are detoxing, even when you are eating blended and live foods (naturally high in water content). Check to make sure that you're drinking from (and optimally even soaking in) a chemical-free water source. Also try to access natural mineral sources if possible, drinking spring water that bubbles up from the earth, or soaking in hot springs. Look online to see what sources might be near you.

Q: I have a question regarding the morning Liver Kick. I tried it twice and in both cases it was very hard for me to drink. My body was completely repelled by the taste and texture. I do want to give my liver the "kick" he needs, so what can I do?

A: You can cut the lemon part of the Kick with an orange or grapefruit. Or try blending with some organic strawberries or blueberries. You may even add some organic raw honey. Drink, enjoy, and try colon hydrotherapy.

As your liver gets cleaner, your aversion to the taste of the Liver Kick will likely go away. The sour from the lemon is what best flushes the liver, so think of it as a very helpful and honest friend who might take some time to get to know, as it pushes buttons in the beginning of your relationship. You may ultimately grow to love this friend.

Also, remember to let your ultimate potential call you forward and make sense of why you're doing this. And know that cleansing gets easier (and more joy inducing) the more you do it.

ACKNOWLEDGMENTS

You cannot teach a man anything; you can only help him to find it within himself. —Galileo Galilei

Anything that comes to us is not truly ours anyway. The manifestation of this book is a culmination of too many experiences and teachings from people that I don't have room to mention here. Yet, as I dig down with the intention of providing the world a gift that is worthy of the time, paper, ink, and people that it will require, I know that I am a conduit and will perhaps receive the credit for this work. I pray it will be as effective for you as it has been for me and the people I've shared it with thus far. Within the endless hours invested, I have realized that this is in fact a labor of love and passion because of the same emotions that I have for all of you, my community, and people of the earth. CNN said a little while back that we "ate our way into this mess and we can eat our way out," but we know that's only a piece of the puzzle, which we will remember in the pages that lie ahead. If you're reading this, I thank you, and if I have ever met you, I thank you, and if you've already participated in this program or any other program I have shared, I thank you. We have all created this somehow together, and I thank you.

There truly is no "I" in "team" and this, like any project, has had many people's attention in order for it to be. Thank you to Anthony J.W. Benson for your care, attention, and stewardship. Thank you Debra Evans for graceful knowledge and beautification. Thank you, Lindsay Sánchez, for all your care and patience in the design process. Thank you, Cher Paul and Sheridan McCarthy, for helping us look better. Thank you so very much to Mouth PR, especially Justin Loeber and Patrick Paris, for all the phone calls and emails that help us deliver this program into the world. Also a very special thank you to my dear friend, Jon Morrow, for being an incredible artist and angel in the design process, as I I really know that if I have your love and okay, that it truly will be so. Thanks also to the amazing Kameko Kali and Marcos Zumaya for the special gardening and research of this program. Also thanks to Sarah Womer, Monet Euan, and Alex Westmore for *The 21-Day Cleanse* beginnings and for knowing and helping it become what it has become, and your support in its service to the world. Thank you to Jessica Unamuno, a great designer and a wonderful addition and support to our team. Lastly, a special thanks to Leelu Morris for having a magical way with images and saving the day a couple times.

To the smartest and kindest man I know, my husband, Michael Karlin, who taught me about many virtues in action, most especially charity, faith, dedication, patience, commitment, and love: thank you for sharing your integrity, structure, and the paradise that is our life with my family and me. Thank you to the amazing Kaplan, Jonas, Smith, Tracy, Ullner, Rivers, Feldstein, Nirgo, Bolno, Segal, Acosta families. Special thanks to D. Soloman and everyone who has made this new chapter of our life so fresh and exciting.

To my family tree and anyone I know of or do not who was part of us becoming. Thank you for your kindness, Aunty Dominique, Bjorn, and Scout, and my dear, wise aunt Rachel Tufunga. Life would not have been the same without the love and hard work of my grandfather Morton Smookler, for whom I am eternally grateful. To all my ancestors and relatives all over the world, I thank you. To my big sister, Sunflower, who paved the way to individuality when I was five, and my sweet brother-in-law, Mitch Stegall, and my precious niece and nephew, Luna and Solwyn. To my spiritual father, Howard Wills, and our beautiful extended family, Ahava and Ramana. Thank you all for enriching our lives again and again.

Thank you to my godparents, Dr. Light and Dr. Bryan Miller, whom I lived with in the glorious Hawaiian Islands as I literally "found myself" in the quiet moments on that Molokai beach at fifteen. Thank you to my other families, the Segalls, for continuous magic and support—Morgan, Scott, and Becci—for making me feel welcome as well as teaching me how to edit and make movies as a preteen, and the McLaughlins for taking me in as well.

All of your homes as well as my own nourished and helped raised me to become exactly who I am today. A special thanks to the glorious nature of Boulder, Colorado, that helped shape me as a child with the Hay, Siegel, Getches, Barish, Balis, and Yaeger families. My mother says it takes roots and wings, and you've definitely been part of the roots.

On the subject of roots, I would also like to thank a few more people who played a profound part in my growth as a human being and indirectly contributed to the life of this project. Thank goodness for my best friends and their reflections through life; they have inspired me in countless ways. I will continue to learn from you always. To the beautiful and dear Lilakoi Moon, amazing songstress Cree Summer, heart-filled activist Josie Maran, beauty queen Leonor Varela, ever-harmonic Donna De Lory, talented Greg Cipes, awesome friend Esai Morales, sweeter-than-sunshine Jennifer Hoffman, Wonder Woman, one-in-a-million Blythe Metz, David Karr, father of Jade, Carlo Marzano, always funny Brian Coletti, family man Ari Chazanas, organic farmer Christopher Daugherty, funny Spiro Palmer, and sweet Dr. Eric Dorninger. It was really fun to roll through life with the imaginary games we invented with our mischievous personalities, always devoted to healing. Thank you for making up many special chapters in our story called life.

Wholehearted thanks to the exquisitely talented Woody Harrelson, and of course my dear friend Brett Harrelson; you both changed my life from my first day on set and inspired me forever. Thanks for gifting me a copy of *Fit For Life* and for a number of other things you introduced me to, including the Santa Monica stairs, Power Yoga, the O2 Bar, and late-night dancing, impromptu yoga sessions at wild parties, the Newsroom Café, looking up at the Maui stars, singing Beatles songs, and living-food birthday cakes!

On that note, I must thank all the greats who helped me even consider the view that we can and perhaps should shine bright without fear to emanate and reflect the stars that we are. The title of the book and all that it encompasses, *The 21-Day SuperStar Cleanse*— "SuperStar" meaning pure light, without holding back, falsifying, or blocking—has been inspired by my life experiences, and I thank you for inspiring me. A warm and special thanks to James Cameron, whose words are like gold in my life and whose commitment to this planet astounds me. Thank you Jason Olive and Lewis Smith and everyone who is a part of the Actors Academy, which warmly lets me contribute. Thank you for your honest support, dear Liz and Bryan Murphy and insightful Charles Mezure. I will always be touched by your teachings. Dearest gracious Janet Yang, awe-inspiring Milos Forman, and smile maker Oliver Stone, thank you for trusting me and changing the course of my life. To my hilarious friend and director Crispin Glover, who cast me as a nun, and all-seeing Thomas Miklautsch, and depth-catching Richard Pichler, who brought me to the Amazon to film and changed my life forever through events I could never explain. To the ever-supportive Michael Davis, fun-loving Terence Michael, committed Richard Salvatore for throwing a ball on set with me. To the Zen David Nakahara, funny Justin Zackham, quick Andrea Ambandos, elevating Mikki Willis, and beautiful Nadia Salamanca for challenging me to stretch even further and for your supportive knowledge and attention on sets. Special thanks to the thousands of people who have been a part of the many productions I have had the privilege of working on and with. I am in awe of all the important pieces of these amazing puzzles. Thank you!

A special thanks to the amazing Kajsa Vikman and everyone who is a part of Lionsgate and BeFit who is allowing us to share free content with the world. Thank you, "fourth-wall remover" Cal Pozo and Sean Kisner for the introduction on that plane ride home from Sundance. Thank you to my guides and artists: I totally respect all that you are and do, genius Philippe Caland and storyteller David Bushelle. Thank you to the writer of Seven Sisters, Raven Cruz, and the lovely Tsa Tsa for letting me see myself in you. Thank you brilliant one, Sean Stone, and the passionate commitment of Heather Rae and the Freedenbergs for helping us see ourselves. Also grateful to my teachers Janet Alhanti and Iris Klein, who never miss a beat, as well as the enthusiastic Jeremiah Comey and Clay Banks for all your authentic guidance. I am in awe of your mastery, Cathi Elliot, Cathi Bosco, and everyone at Landmark including Harris Rappaport and Bryce Brecheisen for your empty and meaningless direct pathway into transformation.

To all the superstars I've been so lucky to work and spend time with. I would never have called myself a teacher, but that's how I continue to learn about these countless lessons, and serving has been an incredible gift. Mind- and body-bending Flea, lord of music Rick Rubin, hilarious Owen Wilson, grounded Peter Berg, philosophical David Duchovny, sweetest Ben and Christine Stiller, heart-flowing, all-knowing minister Jason Mraz, magical David DeLuise, the Marciano family, Eric Etebari, Kingpin, Brent Bolthouse, and the fearless Jared and Shannon Leto along with the band 30 Seconds to Mars and the focused Jeremy Piven. It was a lesson-filled, exciting ride. I am honored to have connected in the light of healing even once, as I was touched by your brilliance, lovely Ashley Olsen, stunning Brooke Shields, otherworldly

Penelope Ann Miller, brilliant John Cusack, and coolest Eric Balfour. Thanks for showing up and supporting my classes (the few that I taught publicly), filmmaker Stevie Long and musical muses Debi Nova, Jillian Speer, and Annalise Bryan—you are all so talented. Thank you sweeter-than-normal Karina Calvert Jones and rare gentlemen Bruce Harrison.

Thank you to a few potent yogis and living Hollywood game changers who deserve a special shout-out, including powerhouse Tara Guber, yoga stud and filmmaker Anthony Mandler, the deliciously bold Kelli Nash, and fashion activist Beth Doane. Thanks to the sound healers Alex Theory, Evolutional Evolve, and the Shriver family. Thank you dear "maha happy yogis" Tom Morley and Steve Ross for making me laugh and being there for us all.

To all the students who came to practice and play with me—you are also my teachers: Natalia, Branca, M'Le, Krista, Taylor, Magda, Ann Levine, Timea, Orsi, Jen, Eliza, Tibaut, Lauralee, and anyone I don't have room to list here. A special thanks also to the lovely Parisian beauties and dearest friends Samantha Panagrosso, Leila Abel, gorgeous Dolores Chaplin, Nora Arnezeder, and Radu Milhanieu for our times doing yoga and being in Cannes.

While on the subject of teachers, I am so lucky to have been able to practice with, learn from, and teach alongside true yogis: like a father, Chuck Miller, like a mother, Maty Ezraty, beautiful Sean Corn, and deep Julie Kleinman. Thank you to the miracle worker Richard Freedman, evolutionary K. Pattabhi Jois, leader Angela Farmer, exquisite Lisa Walford, and everyone at YogaWorks, then and now, including the lovely Sonya Cottle, healer Jasmine Lieb, luminous Shiva Rea, Zen Saul David Raye, shining Kathryn Budig, inspirational Simi Cruz, aligning Paul Cabanis, yoga diva Maryam Askari, and pure Kia Miller. Also thanks to Brother Jay Co, innovative Cameron Shayne, peaceful Rodney Yee, and fierce Duncan Wong. Nothing I practiced or shared would have been the same without the gifted John Friend and *kula*, Amy, Michael, and Sianna: I love you all. Tara Stiles, Ally Hamilton, Bryan Kest, Steve Walter, David Life, Sharon Gannon, and Russell Simmons, thank you for being you and serving in this world.

The pictures in this book and elsewhere have been made possible by the blessings and vivid eyesight of the following talented people: Jeff Skeirik, Craig Cameron Olsen, Leelu Morris, Eliza Balis, Jolie Kinga, Richard Salazar, and James Wvinner—*you are all so talented!* Working with artists like you has truly provided some of the highlights of my life.

Thank you for showing a side of me that I would not know existed without you being there to capture it. To all of you who helped me create art in this life: David Paul, Jeff Boxer, Malibu Mike, Germany Alex for adidas, shooting queen Eliza Balis, cutting-edge Cesario Montano, discoverer David Haskell, English star Leelu Morris, infamous Andy Katz, and too many more to list.

Even beauty is a team effort. Thank you, Hope Zarro and Martine LeBlanc for the hours we've spent making art. To my Israeli queens of beauty, Yonat and Iris at Aesthetics, for giving the best facials ever. To Nurse Jaime and all the girls at Beauty Park and to Jessica Wu, for the book *Feed Your Face*. To my healers and doctors, Dana Shwartz, Carla Farmulara, acupuncturist Boaz Britzman, goddess-loving Bob Ramey, healing-hands Derek Cardoza, clairvoyant Kevin Dowling, ever-present adjuster Bill Domke, and Yoda hands Dennis and everyone at Peak Wellness. To the devotee Indira, lovely Leah, and all those at Clear Way to Health. To the other-worldy rock star healer, Sat Hari Khalsa, beauty maker Marianna Zimmerman, hair genius Marti Perez and Linda Lu.

In regard to all the great business people around me who did their best to provide structure for a bit of a rainbow, I thank you and see the challenges you may have had. Dear Alan Sacks for sage counsel and detailed attention, I am so grateful. Michelle Council, your clarity inspires me, thank you for all. Lon Rosen, for your support along the way. Thank you to Jeff Bennet at SAG, the exceptional trademark attorney Leigh Augustine. Deep thanks to the lovely Hilary Polk William for your time and presence, and to the dear Robert Flutie for your understanding and insight and Michael Flutie for your support with adidas and more. Big thanks to Robyn Klein for being truly so precise. Also to Michael Greenwald, my first but no longer agent, who taught many important lessons.

Giant thanks to all of you at adidas who were a fundamental part of my growth in applying this body of work to myself and sharing it with the world. Thanks to Jim Latham and Jocelyn Robiot for your global support and giving me the opportunity of a lifetime. To Nikki of Pura Vida for your honest reflection. My very special and endless love for Barbara Edisberger and Claire Midwood; you two mean the world to me. To everyone involved with us on the adidas women's line and my signature line, there are too many to mention, but I will always love and be grateful that we got to work together.

Huge thanks to all the journalists who have supported our message in the world by either talking about me or have me on. *The View,* E!, Style, KTLA, *Good day LA, Joan Knows Best,* CNN, *Inside Edition, W Magazine, In Touch, Star, Shape, Details, Natural HEALTH, Cosmo, Fitness, Elle, WWD,* and so many more. Thank you *Yoga Journal, Healing Retreats and Spas, Natural Solutions, Elephant, Body and Soul, LA YOGA,* and *Oxygen Magazine* for your extra attention and cover stories from the beginning. Thank you *Good Day Colorado, Great Day San Antonio, AM Northwest Portland,* Fox, *San Diego Living,* Studio 4, Fashion TV, ESPN, San Fran's *View from the Bay.* It has been a fun and epic adventure getting to spend time with you.

In the realm of PR training, along with all the amazing people with Global PR for adidas, I want to thank Katy Saeger and Marci Mollins as well as anyone else who helped me in a whirlwind of activity. Huge thanks to Elissa Buchter; it was wild, and I totally adore you. Thanks to Anthony Mora and Sharon House for your support in PR at the very beginning. I also need to give a special thanks to Aaron Amid, Felicia Tomasko, Waylon Lewis, Kathryn Arnold, marketing genius Bill Ganz, and everyone who taught me a thing or two about the world including Holly McKay, Fanny Kiefer, Marc Bailey, and Paul Mireles.

In regard to wings, I want to now move into the beloved people I surround myself with nowadays who have changed who I am and given me my wings, and are teaching me to remember what I came here for. Dearest and beloved Juan and Ciela Ruiz, you are my teachers. I am grateful to be able to walk in your footsteps and for all the profound unfolding lessons that you share so masterfully from the heart—infinite thanks. In the vein of my spiritual teachers, I must also thank the entire *la familia*: the Englehearts, the Flores family, Navarros, Davidoffs, Yurie Ann Cho, Heiro Frasheski, Jon Marro, Rory Freedman, Dana Schwartz and David Watts, Jezzerei and Eric Baumgartner, the Hortons, Caroline Kane, Fred and Michaela Kramer, Ben and Ione Lee, Margaret Boll, and Josh Radnor. May we all spread our wings and fly. I want to thank you for your honest reflection and for inspiring me to be better, purer, and more awake.

Also part of this family but with a special bow of my head to your feet, to the deep and all-inspiring devotional music and mastery that you share with us. Thank you Alex and Rosa Cigolini and my beloved sister and brother Avasa and Matty Love. Also on music, thank you dearest Krishna Das and Jai Uttal. Thank goodness you are in this world at all, and I am blessed to know you personally. We have to live and love in the music.

Last but possibly the furthest from least, I am eternally grateful to you, Gurumayi, for your wisdom, beauty, and your clear and direct teachings. Thank you, Your Holiness the Dalai Lama, for your endless service and inspiration. To Mother Teresa for your compassion. To the Hare Krishna temple for your boundless service. To Ammachi, for your hugs and abundant giving. The teachings of *The Urantia Book*, the Kaballah, the Bible, and my time at Shambhala Sun Camp. Thank you to Gandhi for your powerful and life-changing stand. Thank you to Moses for inspiring greatness. To Buddha for creating teachings by example that continue to live on as guidance systems, and a special thanks to the Cosmic Christ and to Krishna who guide us, reminding us always of our path of awakening and remembering.

REFERENCES

HEALTHFORCE NUTRITIONALS
Hard-core vegan organic superfoods
www.healthforce.com

DIVINE ORGANICS BY TRANSITION NUTRITION
Solutions to benefit humankind
www.divineorganics.com

SUNWARRIOR
Transforming the planet one warrior at a time
www.sunwarrior.com

ULIMANA
Primitive chocolate
www.ulimana.com

HOT RAWKS BY RAW-NATION
Organic libido enhancer
www.hotrawks.com

SHAMAN SHACK HERBS
Herbal formulations drawn form a 5000-year-old Pre-Taoist health lineage called The Gate of Life
www.shamanshack.com

LIVING LIBATIONS
Renegade beauty skin care line
www.livinglibations.com

JOSIE MARAN COSMETICS
Luxury with a conscience
www.josiemarancosmetics.com

RAINBEAU MARS LIFESTYLES
Serving the planet one home at a time
www.rainbeaumarslifestyles.com

RAINBEAU MARS OMNIMEDIA
Serving stories that inspire, transform, and heal
www.rainbeaumars.com

DEEPER WELL PUBLISHING
Exploring the depths of health, consciousness, & spirituality
www.deeperwellpublishing.com

GLOBAL GREEN USA
Helping the people, the places, and the planet in need
www.globalgreen.org

RECIPES INDEX

INDEX

*Note: recipes have **bold** page numbers*

ABOUT THE AUTHOR

From her birth under a double rainbow to her rise on the big screen, this actor, author, and innovator has left imprints of her inspiring story around the world. With an irresistible glow, Rainbeau motivates and heals every time she steps into a room. She has a natural ability to guide individuals on a journey to a greener, healthier lifestyle. From her numerous magazine publications, onscreen appearances, and now this book, there is a way for everyone to benefit from Rainbeau's wisdom and nurturing spirit.

In 1996, Rainbeau debuted as an actress in her first feature film with director Milos Forman, a winner of two academy awards. She continued to appear and star in films, television, and videos while also hosting festivals and being the spokesperson for live events. Presently, Rainbeau is cast to star in the upcoming independent film, *Marc & Cleo* from HyperSigil Films.

She is also developing, cowriting, costarring, and coproducing a high-concept feature film, *Seven Sisters*. Staying busy both in front of and behind the camera is Rainbeau's way of using every outlet to serve and deliver inspirational stories.

As an author, her most recent venture is *The 21-Day SuperStar Cleanse*, which shares how to achieve optimal vitality with food, thought, and beauty disciplines. The book is based on her global revitalization program, the 3-Week Cleanse, which is offered seasonally to her online community. Combined with her yoga series on Lionsgate BeFit Channel, and the catalog of twenty full-length workout DVDs and virtual fitness downloads, Rainbeau models her ideal regimen of how health, beauty, and indulgence can coexist, as achieved with thousands of her clients from around the world.

Rainbeau served as the face of adidas women from 2007 to 2009 as their Global Ambassador. During this time she helped develop adidas TV, numerous videos, teacher trainings and manuals, and clothing lines—including her own sold-out sustainable signature clothing line. She traveled to dozens of countries around the world, taught crowds of up to 3500 people, and lead press conferences.

Rainbeau's yoga experience began by teaching A-list celebrities. She was then hired to coproduce, write, and star in what has now become over twenty fitness and yoga video programs that have sold over two million copies around the world.

Rainbeau's 2005 innovation, Rainbeau Mars Lifestyles (RML), now under the umbrella of 2012 Rainbeau Mars Omnimedia (RMO), aims to develop, produce, and deliver stories that inspire, transform, and heal with entertainment through adventurous action and enlightening plots.

Rainbeau is the daughter of author and master medical herbalist, Brigitte Mars. Rainbeau's expertise in health and yoga took shape throughout her teenage years in Molokai, Hawaii, with godparents, Dr. Light Miller, an Ayurvedic naturopath, and Dr. Bryan Miller, a chiropractor. After apprenticing with yoga gurus Chuck Miller and Maty Ezraty as well as many other amazing yoga teachers, Rainbeau began her daily practice of letting go of who she had become to be who she really is.